THE
SPARTAN
WAY

THE
SPARTAN
WAY

**Eat Better · Train Better
Think Better · Be Better**

JOE DE SENA

Founder of SPARTAN RACE

with Jeff Csatari

St. Martin's Griffin ✖ New York

THE SPARTAN WAY. Copyright © 2018 by Spartan Race, Inc. All rights reserved.
For information, address St. Martin's Press, 175 Fifth Avenue,
New York, N.Y. 10010.

www.stmartins.com

Library of Congress Cataloging-in-Publication Data

Names: De Sena, Joe, 1969– author. | Csatari, Jeff, author.
Title: The spartan way : eat better. train better. think better. be better. / Joe De
    Sena, founder of Spartan Race with Jeff Csatari.
Description: First edition. | New York : St. Martin's Griffin, 2018.
Identifiers: LCCN 2018018749 | ISBN 9781250350176 (hardcover) |
    ISBN 9781250153227 (ebook)
Subjects: LCSH: Health. | Exercise. | Mind and body. | Self-care, Health.
Classification: LCC RA781 .D41236 2018 | DDC 613.7—dc23
LC record available at https://lccn.loc.gov/2018018749

Our books may be purchased in bulk for promotional, educational, or business
use. Please contact your local bookseller or the Macmillan Corporate and
Premium Sales Department at 1-800-221-7945, extension 5442, or by
email at MacmillanSpecialMarkets@macmillan.com.

First Edition: September 2018

P 1

DEDICATION

This book has been a culmination of all the experiences and people I have met throughout my life. I want to thank my family, my dad, mom, aunts, uncles, cousins, and close friends. I would be nothing without my wife and the four beautiful kids she brought to us. I also want to thank all of Spartan. The employees, contractors, and all of the community that inspire us to be better.

THE SPARTAN SECRET: THE 11th PRINCIPLE

Good news and bad news.

You're about to learn the Spartan Way. The time-tested principles that have transformed the lives of millions of men and women around the world for thousands of years. You're now starting your own journey.

Before you go, I have a piece of advice for you. There's one more bag to pack for your trip. Frankly, you can't succeed without it. It's indispensable. It was brought to my attention when I was presenting these 10 principles to a special forces group in Fort Bragg, North Carolina. A hand went up in the back of the room.

"Haven't you forgotten something, Joe?"

I had. It was obvious to me in that moment that if there's a single most important secret to transforming your life, this is it. And I'd forgotten to mention it. You might also understand why I and so many forget this most critical principle to achieving success.

You'll find that secret here: life.spartan.com/secret.

CONTENTS

Contents

THE SPARTAN WAY

Human beings thrive on challenge. This has been true for hundreds of thousands of years. It was certainly true for the ancient Spartans. The legendary Greek warriors built the first democracy and one of the finest of militaries on the foundation of a rigorous training program known as the *agoge*. This system turned boys into fierce and loyal fighters through a strict moral code and physical ordeals designed to develop endurance and pain tolerance.

Challenge drives great accomplishment. I've seen it transform lives. But most Americans are way out of practice. We rarely challenge ourselves anymore. Instead, what do we do? We constantly try to make our lives easier, which only makes us weaker and we whine about even the most minor inconveniences. Think about it: You drive a half mile for a quart of milk instead of walking. You swallow mostly processed, heat-and-eat food because you're too busy to cook a healthy meal. You spend more than half of your waking hours sitting. One-third of us are obese. Diabetes is now a worldwide epidemic. Avoiding anything a little bit challenging and uncomfortable has turned us into plush-toy versions of ourselves—soft, overstuffed, and passive.

That seems pretty pathetic to me. So I created Spartan with the goal of ripping 100 million people off their couch cushions. To take action and start living instead of being passive observers.

Look, life is tough. You've just gotta be tougher. You cultivate resilience by facing challenges, not by ignoring them and hoping they'll go away. There are no shortcuts to get to anyplace worthwhile. So my question is: "Are you just gonna lay there with Doritos crumbs on your shirt or are you the kind of person who gets knocked down but gets back up?"

This book, like every Spartan Race, is a rebellion against a life of passivity and softness. It is a rebirth of grit. And it kicks off by forcing you to identify a purpose for your life that'll ignite a fierce, unstoppable passion in you.

This book's purpose is to teach you how to apply the ten timeless principles of the Spartan Lifestyle. If you master these, the next time you're up against the wall, you'll find a way to push through. You'll see. *The Spartan Way* is the ultimate recipe for success. It'll help you embrace adversity and beat any difficult challenge to a pulp.

Tackle it. Own it. We ALL need it.

PREFACE

The heights by great men reached and kept
Were not attained by sudden flight,
But they, while their companions slept,
Were toiling upward in the night.

—HENRY WADSWORTH LONGFELLOW,
THE LADDER OF ST. AUGUSTINE

Chris Davis weighed 696 pounds when we met. This guy would get winded walking from his car to his desk. He was eating eight Egg McMuffins per day and drinking two 2-liter bottles of Mountain Dew. That's 2,832 calories before dinner. Chris was not going to live very long. And he knew it.

Gastric sleeve surgery helped him drop 290 pounds, but he wasn't out of the woods. He still weighed four hundred pounds. And then he got into a horrific car crash. This was back in 2012. His vehicle flipped end over end twice, struck several other cars, and shut down Interstate 85 outside of Atlanta. Amazingly, he walked away with nothing more than a bad seat-belt burn and leg bruises. Surviving the accident gave Chris a second chance at life. It was time he woke up and did something about his weight. So I called him and invited him to come out to Spartan HQ, our seven hundred–acre farm in Pittsfield, Vermont.

My wife Courtney and I had created a home for our four kids in Vermont, but we'd also built a farm to promote the Spartan lifestyle and obstacle races that my company puts on around the world. In Pittsfield, we have a two-story red barn for training, a Bikram yoga studio, a general store, pasture-range and free-range cattle, mischievous goats, and a mountain with fifty miles of rugged trails. It's an ideal location to challenge people to push their bodies and expand their minds. Those people include elite endurance racers and the kind of supermen and super-women who have twenty-plus Ironman races under their belts. But they also include "mortals" like Chris who are in desperate need of a change.

Chris was grateful for the invitation. His employer granted him a leave of absence. With his family's blessing, he drove alone from Atlanta to Pittsfield to spend six months with us. When he arrived, Chris said he had a dream: He wanted to fit into one airline seat when he left and to get ready for the Spartan Ultra Beast, our twenty-six-mile race that contains more than sixty obstacles. That's what he told me. But I knew this man was really in a fight for his life.

"You've just signed up for twenty-six weeks of hell," I told Chris. "Give me your car keys. The only way you're going to succeed is if you're stuck here, so I need your keys and all the money you have on you."

He handed over the keys and his money. In exchange, I handed him a forty-five-pound sandbag. It would become his constant companion throughout the Spartan X training schedule I put together for him. The mental and physical challenges of Spartan X are based on the ten Spartan principles in this book. My job as Chris's instructor was to ignite a bonfire under his ass.

The first day, I had Chris up at 5 a.m. for a ten-mile hike up our mountain carrying his sandbag. We repeated the hike at 5:30 p.m. Same sandbag. It took us hours. Chris was shattered. He'd never walked so far in one go, let alone while hefting a heavy sandbag. Back at home base, I showed him how to toss the sandbag. Then I made him to do it again. And again. And again. His arm and back muscles screamed. Sweat ran in rivers down his chest. His face contorted in pain, but he was feeling something else, too, something that he hadn't felt in a very long while—possibility.

At first, I gave Chris only apples to eat. His system had to clean itself out from all the garbage he'd been consuming. For years he'd lived on fast-food meals, candy, sugary cereals, and soda, all highly processed foods filled with chemicals and preservatives. After a week, I began introducing other raw fruits and vegetables into his diet. He was going through withdrawal, just as an alcoholic or drug addict would in detox. We had to take it slow to get his metabolism back in working order.

Each morning, Chris walked the fifteen hundred stone steps that stretch a mile on the side of our mountain. After his walk, we'd practice kung fu. I had Chris chopping wood and doing yoga. He carried timber and cement bags back and forth until he couldn't see straight. The guy trained like an elite athlete, four to six hours a day, seven days a week.

It wasn't just about building up his physical strength. He was also building up his mental endurance. Tell someone to do thirty reps of push-ups or run five miles and they're already anticipating the finish line. It's well defined. You know what to expect. It's much harder when the endpoint is unknown—it changes the game. When you tell someone to chop wood without stopping or hike up and down a mountain—a distance he can only guess at—he's either going to crash and burn or find the psychological fortitude to endure. The trick is to bring him as close to breaking as you can in order to help him see the power in that psychological grit. We even made Chris write his own obituary. It's sort of a mind game to force him to articulate what he hopes his legacy will be. You'll have a chance to try that exercise at the end of chapter 1.

Chris dragged himself, stunned and beaten, from one challenge to the next. He impressed me. He tackled everything I put in his way. And I could see the changes in his body. He was getting lean and gritty.

This wasn't all about dragging tree trunks up a mountain, 24/7. Being Spartan is about being strong, not stupid. You should train hard but not hurt yourself in the process. Rest and stress relief are important parts of being healthy. Chris learned relaxation techniques, mindfulness, belly breathing, and yoga. The ten-hour hikes helped him sleep better than he'd ever slept before. Swimming in our freezing cold lake horrified him at first. But after a while, I think he craved the feeling of rejuvenation in his sore body.

There were other Spartans at the farm that he hung out with. They almost always ended up in some sort of obstacle competition, like spear throws or burpee challenges. Once a Spartan, always a Spartan.

Chris weighed 262 pounds at the end of his twenty-six weeks on the mountain and nailed the Spartan Beast on Killington, Vermont. That's thirteen-plus miles and thirty obstacles. He flew home sitting in one airline seat.

Just before he left, I caught a glimpse of Chris climbing on the top of the cargo nets obstacle at the farm. He paused on top, smiling and looking off at the mountaintops. Later, I asked him about it. He said he was thinking about how far he had come. He couldn't quite believe he was here and happy to be doing all this crazy shit when just a few months ago there were so many dark moments dragging down his life.

Albert Einstein said that adversity introduces men or women to themselves. I have to believe that Chris got to know himself very, very well during his time with us. He knows what he's capable of now. He's a regular Spartan racer who inspires others. He learned that there really are no limits, only possibilities.

TRANSFORM YOUR LIFE

No matter how far you have gone on a wrong road, turn back.
—TURKISH PROVERB

Even if you're on the right track, you'll get run over if you just sit there.
—WILL ROGERS

ike everyone, I've had roadblocks in my life. Whenever I faced one of those obstacles, I was very lucky to have somebody grabbing me by the collar and pulling me through. I wrote this book with the intention that it will grab you by the collar, and pull you off the couch so you can learn how to overcome roadblocks, too.

I grew up in a *Goodfellas* neighborhood in Queens, a hotbed for organized crime. Around the dinner table we talked about raviolis, the price of concrete, and who was going to and coming from jail. Jail didn't have a negative connotation in my neighborhood. It was like college.

My dad was a workaholic maniac. He had all kinds of businesses, from pizza places and taxi companies to construction and trucking—you name it. The guy leveraged every dollar he had to purchase the "next thing." That worked for a while. Looking back twenty-five years, I know he would have crushed it, but he got over-leveraged. It taught me a lesson: Leverage works big in both directions.

In the eighties, my father started losing everything. Business was upside down. Houses were getting repossessed. Debt collectors were turning up at the door. My parents started fighting over money, quite literally; mom ended up in the hospital a few times.

I was a rudderless kid, looking for a mentor, and I found one in a neighbor. His name was Joe Massino and he was the head of the Bonanno crime family. Everyone knew him as Joe "The Ear" because he insisted that his men never say his name, for secrecy, but touch their ears when referring to him. I was eleven years old when The Ear he took me under his wing. He said, "Hey, we're going to start a business. You're going to start cleaning pools."

I began with his pool. Then he put me in touch with many of his mob colleagues because he told them they could "trust" me in their backyards. Joe was the big boss of the Bonanno family because John Gotti was having legal troubles through some of these years. Through Joe, I did a lot of legitimate pool work for a lot of infamous wiseguys who were all great to me, including "Little Vic" Amuso (a.k.a. Deadly Don), boss of the Lucchese family. (He's currently serving a life sentence on murder and racketeering charges.)

The first thing Joe "The Ear" taught me was that you had to commit. You had to do what you said you were going to do. If I said I would be at his house at 7:15 a.m. on Saturday, then I had better be there at 7:15

a.m. on Saturday, "or else you could end up under the pool," he said. He was joking, but at my age, I took it as a promise. Commitment was expected. Loyalty, pride of work, keeping your word all meant a lot in our neighborhood, and I learned that from Joe "The Ear."

I was happy to be working as a pool cleaner. I wanted to do something, make money, and get ahead, and doing things for the "bosses" added excitement and motivation. It was cool. My father had always taught me that when you meet someone, think about how you can help him or add value to his life. "Make yourself indispensable," he said. I tried to do that for these guys.

I worked my ass off for Joe and he appreciated it. He had only three daughters, so I became like a son to him. He was a generous man on our block. On the Fourth of July, he would send for a tractor trailer to unload fireworks on the street. It would be like World War II for twelve hours; it was insane.

Joe was amazing at asking questions. He would ask the same question twelve different ways in any conversation, which I guess was his way of triangulating the truth. He taught me the importance of paying attention. He had an incredible memory and knew every license plate on the block. When he saw a new plate, he would ask me if I knew whose car it was. Joe was a mob guy who made some bad choices in his life, but I appreciated how he tried to help a neighborhood kid who needed some direction. One thing he said to me that I'll never forget because it changed me forever: "Joe, you put *your* problems on the table, and I'll put *mine* on the table. I bet you will take yours back."

SO-SO IS UNACCEPTABLE

After my parents' divorce, I moved to Ithaca with my mom, but I was still traveling back to Queens to keep my pool business going. It was becoming pretty successful. I had started to bring in other people to work for me.

My first pool staff was made up of neighborhood kids, and that's when I formed a lot of my opinions about success, failure, and motivation. Many of these kids didn't know what they wanted to do in life, they were depressed, and they couldn't wake up on time for work. I started to think that the problem with society was that people had it too easy. I kept thinking, "Shit, I don't have time to breathe . . . I have so many jobs to do and so much work to get done that I have no time to rest. What's with these kids? Why are they so . . . *soft?*"

In my neighborhood, most people worked hard. They had legitimate businesses, such as pizza places, construction companies, trucking companies. Everyone was awake at 5 a.m. They lived their "brand," always putting in extra effort. In our house, too, "so-so" was unacceptable. If you were going to put up the Christmas lights, then you had better put them up perfectly. If you were going to paint the walls or wax the car, they'd better be perfect. My father used to say, "We measure a quality job in micrometers."

My dad and Joe "The Ear" instilled a strong work ethic in me that helped me on many occasions. I learned the importance of playing like a pro, providing top service. I became relentless at everything. There were no weekends at the beach, there was no time off, no vacations. If the phone rang, you were on the job. If the phone didn't ring, you had better make it ring. I could see the drive for success in the local bricklayers, the pizza-shop owners, the welders, whomever. Those who outworked, out-marketed, outproduced the other guys were the ones who got the jobs. They were always on, and they were crushing it. Thirty-four years later, I realized that the core values I started learning in this neighborhood guided me over every roadblock in my life. I've returned to them time after time and they've helped me achieve every victory I've won, big or small, like finishing a hundred-mile endurance race or building a profitable business. What I found interesting as I began interviewing successful people for our Spartan Up! podcast was that most of them lived by the same set of core values. They are universal.

The Spartan Way is the culmination of a lifetime of real-world lesson learning and the generous advice of others. During my 18,142 days on this earth, I have become convinced that these ten principles and the Spartan Core Virtues define the quintessential blueprint for successful living.

Apply these ten principles, and you'll get through a Spartan Race, start a business, or build a great family. They'll help you to lose a hundred pounds or earn an advanced degree. Just name the goal. *The Spartan Way* will push you to face up to challenges, piss on those self-defeating thoughts that are holding you back, and overcome the gnarliest of obstacles. The principles in this book force you to identify the worst and the best in yourself, and to focus on your goals, so that your first steps turn into many miles that ultimately lead you to your finish line.

Police officers, ex-military, working moms, single fathers, overweight CEOs, students, teachers, dropouts—anyone can benefit from these principles. All you have to do is commit to them and let them 10X your life.

Nelson Mandela once said, "It's your reaction to adversity, not adversity itself, that determines how your life's story will develop." I love that quote because it dumps the responsibility right in your lap, where it should be. Adversity is around every corner. You can't escape it. How you handle that adversity is how you build your legacy.

Look, everybody has demons and challenges to destroy. We are all in the same mud pit. You've taken the first step toward climbing out and moving forward by picking up this book. What'll make you different from everyone else will be how you use your brain, body, and grit to overcome whatever it is you need to overcome. *The Spartan Way* will help you do that.

Each chapter in this book covers a key principle for developing a particular Spartan virtue. There are a lot of words in here, but words can

THE SPARTAN CORE VIRTUES

Through work and endurance racing I have come to know many people. Some of them were unforgettable. These great ones all shared the same core qualities. I call them the Spartan Core Virtues. Combine these qualities into one person and you have the ideal boss, the valuable employee, the perfect business partner, or comrade in any endeavor. Here's a short description of each of the Spartan Core Virtues:

Self-Awareness: Know who you are and who you are not. If you don't, you'll be confused daily.

Commitment: Stick to it because the world is filled with people who don't. You're better than that.

Passion: If you're not passionate about what you do, you're not going to be great at it. Take things seriously and learn to be passionate.

Discipline: Set your rules and stick to them. Be disciplined about it.

Prioritization: Deal with the important things—important being what you define as important—first.

Grit: Get gritty. Break out of your comfort zone. Do the hard, scary shit. Find your passion and persevere.

Courage: This is the ability to stay focused and work relentlessly with both intensity and passion through virtually anything, especially through failure.

Optimism: See the world as you want it to be, not as it is. Be ever hopeful.

Integrity: If you're not honest with yourself and others, then what are you?

Wholeness: Live the life of a complete and whole Spartan.

only take you so far. Only decisive action triggers real change. So I've put together a working plan to help you engage each Spartan principle in your life on a daily basis. These plans appear at the end of each chapter. You can't miss them; they're identified with one of my favorite sayings, "Get Off the Couch!" Don't skip these exercises. They're mandatory, like the thirty burpees you're required to pump out if you can't complete an obstacle in a Spartan Race. Get 'em done.

Why are the exercises so important? Think about the logic here: Mastering a new behavior takes work. Drilling. Practice. You can't read something and *think* your way to change. Change happens only when you make it happen, through doing the hard stuff. Here's an example to help you understand this.

THE COMBAT ROLL

The first skill you want to learn in white-water kayaking is something called the "Eskimo roll." When your kayak flips upside down in the middle of raging rapids (likely to happen sometime), you need a way to flip yourself upright in order to breathe. Your other option is to "wet exit," which means wiggling out of the cockpit like a salamander and then chasing your kayak as it floats downriver (not advised). The Eskimo roll is the better option. Here's how you roll: When your boat flips upside down in the river and your legs and hips are still wedged inside the kayak, you tuck your upper body to the deck of the kayak. Then you sort of bend your torso like a "C" shape and quickly snap your hips outward, which should roll your boat upright. *Should.*

Can you picture it? I didn't think so. You can't learn to perform an Eskimo roll just by reading the instructions. You learn by doing. It's the only way. You practice, first in a pool or lake. And once you've mastered the Eskimo roll in calm water, you practice it in the middle of Class IV rapids. That's where kayakers often have referred to it as a "combat roll" because you perform it in dangerous river conditions, hanging from your upside-down kayak with rocks hitting your helmet and the sharp sting of cold river water up your nose.

See, you have to get off the couch in order to grow. You have to learn the messy way, by doing the hard work. Reaching any goal means, literally, reaching and stretching out of your comfort zone into the turbulent waters of life.

That's what this book is going to help you accomplish. How long will it take? I don't know. But give yourself thirty-six days. I find that a deadline (or a stopwatch) can be a great kick in the ass. Thirty-six days, a little more than a month, is about what it takes for most people to turn

a practice into a habit. If you can commit to following these ten principles for thirty-six days, the Spartan virtues will become part of your core
forever.

So get fired up! You deserve to 10X your life.

—Joe

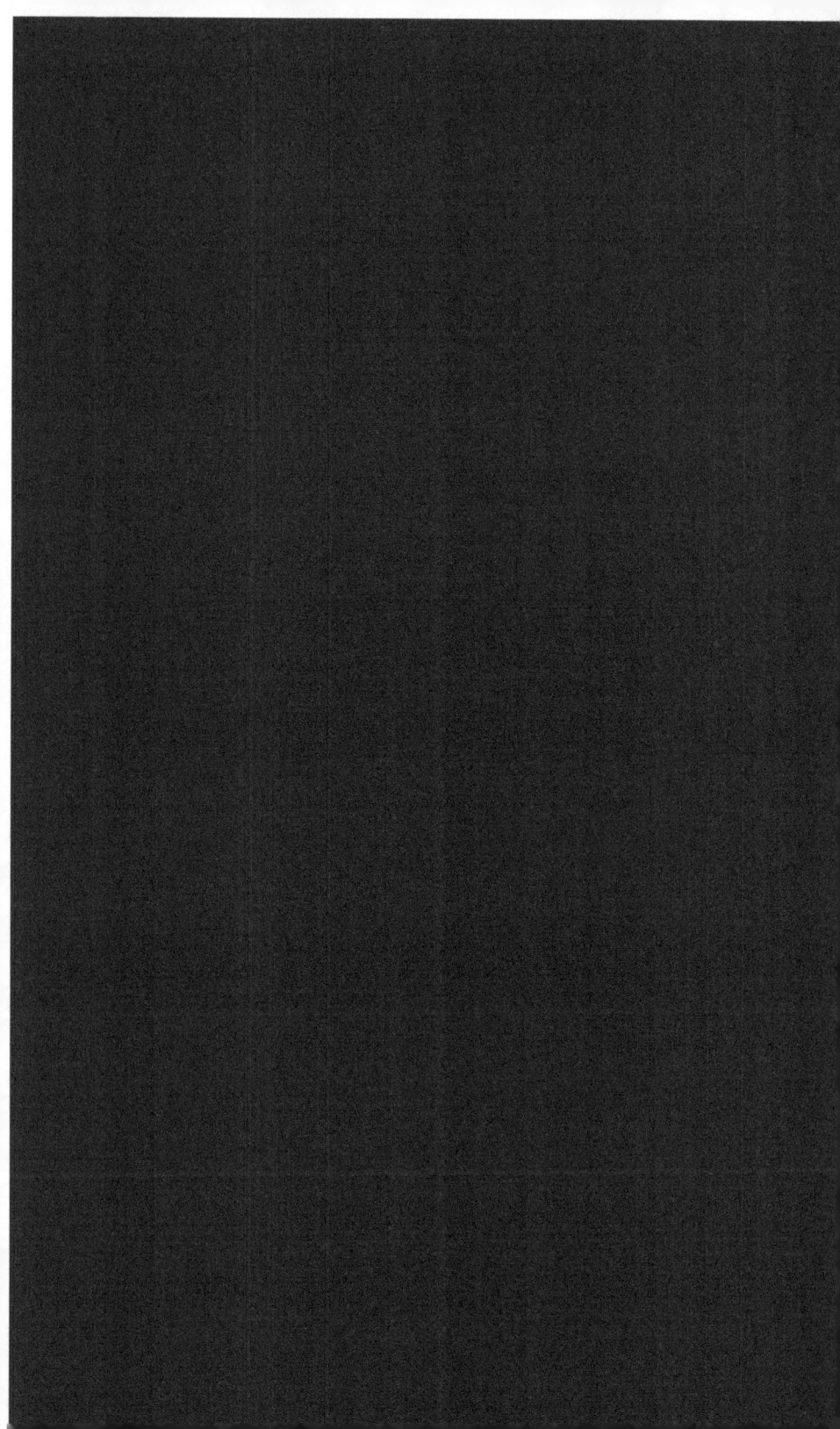

PRINCIPLE #1

FIND YOUR TRUE NORTH

Efforts and courage are not enough without purpose and direction.
—JOHN F. KENNEDY

*Many men go fishing all of their lives without knowing
that it is not fish they are after.*
—HENRY DAVID THOREAU

For millennia, the North Star has helped human beings find their way. People have sailed boundless seas and crossed trackless deserts without getting lost. They had a permanent beacon in the night sky to keep them on track.

Hunt for the North Star the next time you're outside, away from city lights on a clear night. It is easy to find if you can I.D. the constellation Ursa Major, the Big Dipper. The two outer stars in the bowl of the Dipper always point directly to the North Star.

The North Star, also known as Polaris, is a fixture in the night sky, always positioned directly over the North Pole. It neither rises nor sets. It's constant and reliable, which is why it's also referred to as the True North.

Just to be clear and avoid misunderstandings, Magnetic North, where your compass needle points, is about 310 miles away from the True North Pole. Its location shifts several kilometers every year, due to fluctuations in the Earth's magnetic fields.

We're focusing on True North here. Like the North Star, your True North will be an uncompromised beacon that you can always count on to guide you. It's NOT 310 miles shy of your goal. It's spot on. That's why figuring out your True North is the most important Spartan principle.

Have you seen the movie *Hacksaw Ridge*? It was directed by Mel Gibson and it came out in 2016. It's violent, but good and worth renting. It's based on a true story about a World War II US Army private named Desmond Doss who refused to carry a gun into combat.

Doss was a quiet, skinny kid from Lynchburg, Virginia, who'd grown up with a strong faith, using the Ten Commandments as God's direction for how to live his life. As a Seventh-day Adventist, he vowed never to kill or even touch a weapon.

The movie is set in 1942 with the Second World War in full swing and the American body count growing. Even though his religious beliefs were incompatible with war, Doss felt compelled to help his fellow Americans, so he enlisted in the Army. That's not a good place to be if you don't like guns. In boot camp he refused to take target practice and he was severely ridiculed and intimidated, even beaten, by his peers. Officers tried to get him court-martialed.

It didn't work. In the summer of 1944, Doss was deployed with the

307th Infantry, 77th Infantry Division, as a combat medic on Guam in the Philippines. Doss found himself in the thick of the Battle of Okinawa, one of the longest and grimmest engagements of the war. The Allies would lose fifty thousand men, the Japanese more than a hundred thousand.

At one point, the Allies captured the Maeda Escarpment, a jagged four-hundred-foot ridge riddled with Japanese tunnels. But a surprise attack left hundreds of Americans from Doss's unit either dead or dying on the ridge. Doss jumped into action. He ignored orders and sprinted into battle with only his Bible and first-aid box. Over the course of the next five hours, he pulled seventy-five wounded men from the field and lowered them to safety down a cliff using a makeshift pulley system.

That wasn't all. Back in the field to search for more wounded, he took shrapnel from a grenade. While being evacuated, Doss gave up his place on the stretcher when he saw another wounded soldier. While waiting for the stretcher-bearers to return, he was shot by a sniper.

What an amazing story of fearlessness and dedication to a goal. Imagine crawling up and back through mud and a hail of bullets and saving seventy-five guys without ever firing a shot to protect himself.

President Truman awarded Doss the Medal of Honor in 1945. Years later, someone asked Doss why he wouldn't defend himself when he was lying wounded on that bloody ridge. "I knew if I ever once compromised, I was going to be in trouble," he said. "Because if you can compromise once, you can compromise again."

I love that line: "If you can compromise once, you can compromise again." Giving in once makes it easier to give in a second and third time and a fourth. I tell this story because Doss was a man who knew his True North and followed its lead to the end without giving in. No compromise. That's the kind of commitment you need. Your True North goal needs to be worthy of that level of dedication.

Doss is an extreme example, but you've seen people around you with similar laser-beam focus on their goals. People who are following their True North think and act differently than other people do. They have a burning drive that blocks out all the extraneous crap that can be so distracting. People who don't follow a True North are in a very different place. They don't know where they want to go. And if they don't know where they want to go, how in hell can they get there?

Here's the best part about setting your internal GPS on your North Star: It's easy to say, "fuck you" to distractions. True North keeps you constantly moving in the right direction and makes certain you won't somehow stray off course by the pull of other people's agendas. When you own your True North, your life isn't controlled by external factors. Having a True North eliminates indecision and inspires confidence. Why? Because it's well defined and always at the top of your mind. Your True North should make you jump out of bed like a kid on Christmas morning.

WHERE IS YOURS?

Your True North is always inside of you. You just need to find it. It's a fixed point set by your deeply held beliefs and values. And it's drawing you toward one direction. If you fight it, you'll quickly lose your bearings and become lost. Align with it and your True North will act like a high-speed train pulling you through life.

Private Desmond Doss didn't second-guess himself. He followed the pull of his internal compass and became an unlikely hero. We all have the opportunity to become heroes to our partners and kids and our friends and communities if we decide to be guided by our True North. Most important, we can be heroes to ourselves.

But most folks will never get there because they're stuck in the mud of mediocrity. They don't move toward their True North because they either don't know what it is or because they don't fully commit to following it. They're fearful of change and addicted to their comfort zone. These are people who can't tell you what motivates them.

Others have priorities that are ass-backwards. They pursue pleasure at the cost of fulfillment. They're scared of failure, so they never try. They avoid the adrenaline rush of attacking adversity and instead reach for a Red Bull to get through the day. It pisses me off to see people ambling through life without purpose. It's such a frigging waste of time, talent, and potential for making this world a better place to live. That's why it's my personal mission to "get people off the couch" of sedentary complacency and become engaged in life—maybe even for the first time.

Yeah, Joe De Sena can be intense. Some people think I'm a little crazy because of the Death Races and making people carry buckets of rocks up muddy hills. But I'm also wildly optimistic about human potential and our intrinsic spirit. I know there are millions of people who long to get off the couch and start living mindfully and physically. You picked up this book (thanks, by the way), so you obviously see the value in finding and prioritizing your True North. As you read on, you'll see why this first principle is so important.

Use this chapter to re-align yourself with your authentic purpose. You can do it no matter how many years you may have been pulled off course. But you have to *do it* already. No procrastinating. Life is too short to put off something so powerful.

How do you start? With self-awareness. It's the first step on your Spartan journey. It's also one of the hardest to master. Most people go through life on automatic pilot, disengaged and unaware of their authentic desires. Like water flowing downhill, they seek the path of least resistance. They're lazy. Or maybe they simply lack direction, like the kid I was before I met Joe "The Ear."

It has been estimated that we spend half of our waking hours daydreaming, disengaged, unfocused, and unaware of what we're doing. Think about it: That's half of your life! But that's the way we're wired. Unless we do something to break the circuit.

THE BRAIN'S DEFAULT MODE

I've always felt that some people trudge through life like zombies. They walk around looking for stimulation here or there but most of the time they are lost in their thoughts, in a perpetual fog. It's like they're not engaged in life, not aware of what's going on around them.

Well, I was surprised to learn that some folks who are a lot smarter than me have been thinking about this, too. In recent years, neuroscientists have been using fMRI brain scans to explore what's going on when we're not doing much other than just thinking to ourselves or staring off into space during a boring meeting. It turns out our brains are not resting at all but spending a lot of energy on background chatter. Researchers say that, from moment to moment, our brains interact with the world through two types of networks.

One is the direct experience network, when you are experiencing information coming into your senses in real time, like when you're doing the Atlas Carry challenge during a Spartan race. You're not worrying about next week's sales meeting. You're just trying to carry a cement ball without dropping it on your toes.

The second is what neuroscientists call your *default mode network* (DMN), because it engages when not much is going on in the real world and you have the time and space to think about yourself, ruminate about that sales presentation, worry about what your teenagers are doing, or daydream about a vacation. When your brain is absorbed in the default mode network, brain docs say you're creating a narrative using vast stores of memories of people, places, your history, and thoughts of the future. There's nothing critically wrong with this human tendency to space out, but when you spend most of your time lost in the DMN thought, you lose your sense of the present moment and the path to your True North.

It also seems to me like a big waste of time. This is more than just my observation: It is backed up by some big brains at Harvard University. Two psychologists there named Matthew Killingsworth and Daniel T. Gilbert conducted a study using an iPhone Web app to gather 250,000 data points on people's thoughts and feelings as they went about their lives. They made a startling discovery: People spend 46.9 percent of their waking hours thinking about something other than what they're doing. In other words: mind-wandering. Imagine that. Half of our lives are spent spacing out. That is the human brain's default mode of operation. The problem is, Killingsworth and Gilbert say, "A wandering mind is an unhappy mind."

When our minds wander, we usually dwell on negatives. We're jealous of our neighbor's new open-air Fiat 124 Spider. Or maybe we're busy beating ourselves up over events that happened in the past, or we're worrying about the future. None of these brain activities is particularly productive, which is why we need to do a better job of living in the moment.

The first step toward living in the moment is to recognize your personal thinking style. Are your thoughts keeping you from following your True North? See if you identify with any of these unhelpful styles of thought listed in Thinking Bad on the next page.

The path out of the jungle of negative thought patterns is self-awareness. You first need to be aware of when your mind is being hijacked by negative thoughts of past and future. Then you need to fight your way back to the present. Think about all the many philosophical and

THINKING BAD
How Many of These 5 Negative Styles of Cognition Do You Use?

Black-and-white thinking. There are no gray areas. You feel that things are one way or the other, always.

Tunnel vision. You think through a filter, focusing on the negatives and ignoring the positive possibilities. This kind of thinking screws with what is rational.

Minimizing and maximizing. People who tend to think this way often see themselves as inadequate and everyone else as A-list. Facebook fosters this kind of mind game. Nobody posts anything but the best parts of his or her amazing life on Facebook. Here's a tip: Stop comparing yourself to everyone on Facebook. You're only seeing the highlight reel.

Jumping to conclusions. You tend to expect a negative outcome so you foresee a final score before the game's over.

Catastrophizing. You overreact to news, turning smoldering embers into forest fires. Being unrealistic often goes hand in hand with using "never" and "always" statements, such as "He always wins" and "I never catch a break." These are typically generalizations that just aren't true.

When you sense these negative thought patterns creeping into your head, call them out for what they are (lies, lies, lies) and focus instead on your True North.

religious traditions that teach that happiness is to be found by living in the moment.

Next step: With a clear head, actively identify your guiding values. I like to think of my core values as the bull's-eyes of life and my beliefs as the arrows that either hit or miss those targets. For example, if you value being healthy but you believe it's okay to smoke a few cigarettes every day, then you are not going to hit your target, and you're not going to be healthy. If you value family, like I do, but you believe you have to work eighty-hour weeks, including weekends, regularly missing events in your kids' lives, then you're not going to hit that target. If you value becoming your company's top-producing salesperson, but you allow your wandering mind to ruminate on past failures and rejection, it'll be hard to get out of your head and into your next sales call.

To have a clear sight of your True North, you have to be shooting at the right targets with the right arrows at all times. That means aligning your values and beliefs with your daily activities. If you value exercise, you build exercise into your day. If you value community, you find a way to spend time with friends, neighbors, and civic organizations no matter how busy you happen to be.

This is a lot easier to grasp than it is to execute. That's because the brain is a wily organ that can trick us into thinking what we want to think. A famous social psychologist named Leon Festinger developed an idea for why this happens, called the "theory of cognitive dissonance," through his research at the University of Minnesota and Stanford University in the 1950s. Festinger said that we often reinterpret what we do or know to fit more comfortably with what we believe about our world or ourselves. For instance, if you value health, but also love to drink red wine, you might rationalize that drinking two big glasses of cabernet with dinner and a third as a nightcap every day is a healthy practice that won't harm you. You might even seek out information on the internet about the health

---

WHAT I'VE LEARNED

Thom Beers, television producer (THE DEADLIEST CATCH, ICE ROAD TRUCKERS, AND STORAGE WARS), founder BoBCat and Digiland

Life is not a destination, it's just a journey, so in everything you do, do it one step at a time and do it better than anybody else. There's no reason to do anything half-ass. If you're driven you can succeed. Passion is probably the most important thing in the world. If it doesn't make your heart pump Kool-Aid, it's probably not worth doing.

---

benefits of resveratrol, the antioxidant in red wine, to support your "healthy" behavior. If you find yourself defending decisions or behaviors that don't fulfill you or just don't feel right, then cognitive dissonance may be at play. Or you may simply be trying to uphold values that don't ring true to your life.

That's why it's so important to search your soul for your True North. You need to find a passion that resonates so deeply within you that you don't have to think twice. You don't have to force yourself to do what you want and need to do. You're in a zone where you're automatically drawn to the challenge. It's what I call "effortless effort." There's no mistaking when you're in this place. You feel great about the person you've become when you're fully engaged.

Let me give you an example of what I mean through the story of a friend of mine—a former NFL player named Anthony Trucks.

WELCOME THE BATTLE

Trucks's first memory, at age three, is of his mother giving him and his siblings away to a foster family. "During those early years, I remember feeling less than human," he told me. "I experienced physical and mental abuse, starvation and torture." He bounced through several foster families. One of his foster mothers developed MS. As a teen he was arrested at gunpoint. At fourteen, he testified in court to sever his natural mother's rights in order to be adopted. But he started to search for his True North one day in high school English class, when he overheard a girl casually attributing the fact that he was flunking out to his being a foster-care kid. It was a throwaway remark that painfully hit home. He decided there and then that he was not going to fit that label, and that he was not going to use his challenges as an excuse to fail.

In a remarkable reversal, Trucks graduated high school, got a football scholarship at the University of Oregon, earned a degree in kinesiology, and ended up playing two seasons at linebacker for the Redskins and the Steelers before injuries forced him to retire. Today, he's a respected author, high-earning consultant, and proud father of three.

Through football, Trucks discovered his self-worth and purpose and also a burning desire to leave a positive impact on the world. His journey was grueling, but Trucks says, "I fell in love with the enormity of it. There's an ecstasy inside the pain. I like the journey, the battle, the fight, because I feel it tests me every moment of the day, and I love that."

You can find the same kind of drive that Trucks discovered. Start from where you are now. Look at your own values and beliefs. Question what kind of contribution you're making in the world and what you can possibly bring to the table every single day of your life. Ask yourself what journey are you on right now? What direction are you going in? How would you live this day if it were going to be your last? What would you think back on and be proud of? What would you regret? How would your eulogy read if you had lived a long, full life and died of old age?

In the Introduction, I told you that we asked Chris Davis to write his own obituary when he found his way to us on the farm, desperate for change in his life. I want you to do that now, too. What would your obituary read if someone were writing it today? What legacy would you be leaving? You see, your True North is directly related to your legacy. And everything you do, every action you take, every decision you make, must move you forward toward this legacy. Anthony Trucks didn't want his legacy to be that of another forgotten foster kid who just bailed on life.

Once you know what you want your legacy to be, you'll find it directly impacts your beliefs, your values, and, most significantly, the direction you take in life. It will guide you to your True North. If your legacy is to be the greatest marathon runner in the world, you won't quit a race no matter how tired, dehydrated, or broken your body is. If your legacy is to be a great dad, you'll tell your boss, "Sorry, I can't work next weekend," and you'll find a way to get the job done in eight hours instead of fifteen.

Knowing your legacy and reflecting upon it will keep you going in the right direction. In his now legendary 2005 Stanford commencement speech, Steve Jobs said, "Remembering that I'll be dead soon is the most important tool I've ever encountered to help me make the big choices in life. Because almost everything—all external expectations, all pride, all fear of embarrassment or failure—these things just fall away in the face of death, leaving only what is truly important."

What was truly important to Jobs was to put "a ding in the universe." He achieved this through his role as a visionary who completely changed how we communicate and live in the world. That others recognized this

> # WHAT I'VE LEARNED
> **Elizabeth Weil, Managing Director,**
> **137 Ventures, and marathoner**
>
> Everyone should have a small personal advisory board. Those
> people should be peppered from weird spots in your life. So it
> might be an old professor or an old colleague, someone who
> knows you very, very well. Check in with those people and have
> them be your gut check as you go through life.

as his legacy is unquestionable. After Jobs's death, people left flowers in
his memory outside Apple stores around the world. How many CEOs do
you know who'd be honored this way? How many CEOs are household
names? A handful, at best.

Everyone's legacy is different, and whether you want to be an awesome parent, a great athlete, or a hugely successful entrepreneur, it's also
important to know that your purpose in life can change—just as Doss's did
once the war was over. He went on to live a quiet life with his sweetheart.
He never again had to dodge machine-gun fire and put his own life in danger by pulling a wounded man to safety. But he knew he could—and he
would—if he had to.

The problem, as far as I can see, is that close to 99 percent of people
don't know what their purpose is at any stage of their lives. They just drift
toward some fuzzy future goal, relying on comfortable and convenient
choices to get there. If things get tough in the process, they just switch direction or cower in fear. They lack self-awareness; they don't reflect on

their lives. They sweat the small stuff and blame everyone but themselves for their misery.

The remaining 1 percent, though, have figured out their values, and they know the steps they need to take to support them. They know what they want their legacy to be, and they're determined to keep their eyes on the prize and follow their True North.

My question to you is this: Which percentage are you in now? Is it the one in which you want to live?

PRINCIPLE #2

MAKE A COMMITMENT

(SPARTAN VIRTUE: PERSEVERANCE)

If a man hasn't discovered something that he will die for, he isn't fit to live.
—MARTIN LUTHER KING, JR.

If you aren't going all the way, why go at all?
—JOE NAMATH

I take my family to live abroad for an extended time every year. Uprooting a young family is the crazy, logistical hassle you can imagine it is. It would be so much easier to stay home. But my wife Courtney and I have decided to make these trips because we feel so strongly about their benefits. It's a way to immerse ourselves in another culture and gain new perspective on our own lives. These trips also enable me to see the principles guiding this book on a deeper level. Just setting foot on the mountainside in Japan famous for its "Marathon Monks" is an unforgettable lesson in commitment.

Mount Hiei is about twenty kilometers northeast of the ancient city of Kyoto. If you hike in springtime, as we did, the steep trails through dense forest give way to massive fields of blazing azaleas. It's like the Fourth of July in April. A little farther on, lines of towering cedars shelter your path toward the summit. The 848-meter peak blew me away.

I told my family we were going to take a short hike to see an ancient temple. I lied. The temple part was true, but the hike turned out to take about six hours! And I didn't tell them the real reason for the hike: I was grave hunting.

At the top of Mount Hiei there is a Buddhist temple complex called Enryaku-ji that's steeped in history. Several centuries ago, more than three thousand temples dotted this mountain and were home to an army of warrior monks. Now, there are fewer than fifty shrines and stupas, the majority having been burned down by a powerful shōgun in the sixteenth century.

This place has played a central role in the cultural legacy of Japan and it is now a designated world heritage site. The warrior monks are long gone, but it is still home to another badass Buddhist sect known as Tendai-shu: The Marathon Monks.

The Marathon Monks are known for their commitment to one of the most grueling physical and spiritual challenges in human history, the *sennichi kaihōgyō,* which translates to "circling the mountain." Chosen monks embark on epic solo walking meditations around Mount Hiei over a period of one thousand days that are broken into one-hundred-day hikes over the course of seven years. Over time, a monk builds enough endurance to walk more than twenty-six miles a day, the equivalent of a marathon.

After seven hundred days, the monk also begins a nine-day fast; he won't eat, sleep, or even lie down. He'll take just a small cup of water nightly. Then he continues for another 300 days. If he completes the journey, the monk's reward is said to be enlightenment. If he fails to finish, his punishment is death by his own hand. The monk disembowels himself using a knife or hangs himself with a rope. He carries both tools on the journey. The mountain is dotted with many unmarked graves of those who have failed in their quest.

These were the graves I had come to see. I wanted to pay homage to these fallen warrior monks who took their commitment so seriously that they would rather die than live having failed in their quest.

Anyone who knows me understands the importance I place on commitment, the second Spartan success principle. I see very few gray areas here. Commitment is critical to success, yet most people don't know how to commit—or they don't want to commit. They quit too easily or they prefer to be passive observers of life. That's not only bullshit, it's a recipe for failure. If you want to really succeed, you're either all in or not in at all. The Tendai-shu monks knew that before taking their first steps.

Throughout history, only 45 of some 450 monks completed this extraordinary challenge. All, however, believed that they could do it, and they committed to following their True North every single day on that mountain.

Do you know what commitment is? It's a compelling personal promise you make that determines how you will lead your life day to day, moment to moment. The beauty of committing yourself is that it makes the rest of life's decisions easy for you. If you look to your True North for direction, it's easy to say "no" to a cocktail offer, a third slice of pizza, or a meeting that will take you away from a scheduled workout. You can tell the boss "no" to working the weekend without regret because your commitment to family comes first. Do you see now how important identifying your True North is to this second virtue? How completely you commit to your path will determine if you reach your destination or metaphorically disembowel yourself along the way.

MASTER CLASS
Dean Karnazes, the ultramarathoner who ran 50 marathons in 50 states in 50 consecutive days

COMMITMENT

Put some skin in the game. Sign up for an event. Put money on the table. Then email all your friends and say, "I'm running this (marathon) and I'm running it for charity." Pick a charity you admire. And that puts some pressure on you, because when you want to come home and have some pizza and drink a beer, you think, I've got a marathon coming up. So you get after it. Now you're on the hook.

DESPERATE GROUND

When I started endurance racing, I made a pledge to myself that I would always finish the race. No matter the pain I was in, or the discomfort, the fear, the fatigue I might be experiencing, I would complete the race. Whether it was a hundred-mile footrace in the snow or a six-day trek in blazing desert heat, I would prepare, and I would meet the challenge. I would never question how far the finish line might be. I knew I would eventually reach it because I had committed to being that person who finishes the race.

In the ancient Chinese text *The Art of War*, author Sun Tzu called that place where there are no options for retreating or quitting "desperate ground." He wrote: "Throw your soldiers into positions from whence there is no escape and they will prefer death to flight. If they will face death, there is nothing they may not achieve. Officers and men alike will put forth their utmost strength."

How could you create a "desperate ground," where achieving victory is the only acceptable option? No retreat. No quitting. No other option than to persevere.

A friend told me the story of a pastor of a large Presbyterian church who was leading a six-week workshop called "Saving Our Marriage" for troubled couples on the brink of divorce. The first evening, he spent forty-five minutes detailing the physical, psychological, social, spiritual, and financial costs of divorce. Then he handed each couple a contract to take home. It read: "We agree that divorce is not an option and we will do whatever it takes to save our marriage."

"Take it home and pray about it," the pastor said. "Search your hearts. If you cannot commit to taking divorce off the table and committing to doing the hard work that is needed, please do not come back here next week. Good night."

When there is no other option, you will find a way to finish your race, whatever it may be. In my marriage, business, and other important aspects of life, I'm committed to success. It's the strength of that commitment that makes me try harder when faced with obstacles. Problems are always going to crop up. I've decided that I will find a way to hurdle them no matter what. I'm on desperate ground. Fortunately, I have an awesome wife who is equally committed to our marriage, our family, and our collective goals.

Commitments are powerful, and they can make life less confusing by guiding you through tough times of fear and indecision. If you're committed to losing forty pounds, you won't come home every evening, crack open a beer, and spend the next five hours slumped on the sofa surfing through mind-numbing television shows. Your commitment will naturally lead you to get out for a run, cook a healthy meal, or do any number of things that will inch you toward your weight-loss goal.

Commitments require big, uncomfortable feelings, and perseverance. It's true Spartan virtue. The ancient Spartans were unstoppable because of their unifying commitment to one another. They fought and died for each other. They also challenged each other, which deepened the level of their commitment. In the *agoge,* the education and training system that Sparta's boys entered at age seven, fighting was actively encouraged as a means of sorting out spats and squabbles. The brawling hardened them into warriors who respected one another's strength. They knew that when they went into battle, they were among brothers who were equally committed to succeeding.

I signed my boys up for a wrestling camp in Upstate New York. An intensive fourteen-and-under wrestling camp is about as close as a kid can get to experiencing a Spartan *agoge*. Wrestling is just a tough fucking sport. It's no wonder the Special Forces recruit from college wrestling programs.

> Once you've wrestled, everything else in life is easy.
>
> —DAN GABLE,
> Olympic wrestler and gold medalist
> (1972) and legendary head coach
> at the University of Iowa

Most of the kids there had a dad who wrestled. We are not a wrestling family. I didn't really know what to expect, but the camp impressed the hell out of me. These kids are real warriors. They are up at 6 a.m. running two miles, then it's two and a half hours of practice, eat, then another two and a half hours of practice. Repeat. They're going full throttle all day. The kids can barely see straight by the afternoon.

I brought my two boys and my nephew to the camp. One was eleven, the other two were nine. As soon as we got there, I took them to a barbershop to get crew cuts. I figured, these kids are literally going to war from

Sunday to Thursday. They are going to get beat up and I need them to bond to get through this thing. So we got crew cuts and we had some Chipotle and they went into battle. I'm proud of those guys. They got their asses whupped, shed a tear here and there, but never quit.

Over the years of running Spartan Races, I've seen so many people quit during an event. Sometimes they drop out very near the starting line when they're faced with carrying a thirty-pound sandbag across a river and up a hill. Other times it happens just a short distance from the finish line. They pull up and shrug, and say something disappointing like, "Well, at least I tried," or "I gave it my best."

Why do they quit? They quit because at that moment they want to quit. It's easier to say, "Fuck this. I'm outta here!" than it is to go on. But here's something else that is crucial to understand: Quitting is easy for them because they allowed themselves that option before they even started. A commitment is half-hearted if you've already green-lighted a bail option in case of "emergency." The Marathon Monks had a rope and dagger to remind them of the insane seriousness of their commitment. Sun Tzu advised sending warriors to battle on "desperate ground" where retreat was not an option. Joe De Sena's vehicle would not become a getaway car for three boys at wrestling camp.

Where will you find your motivation to push on when every aching fiber of you wants to quit? Your answer is in chapter 1. Once you have identified your True North and defined your legacy, commitment is the logical next step. Like the monks, you'll start your journey believing you are capable of making tremendous things happen. That, however, means you need to do something that most of us have huge difficulty with: being completely honest with yourself.

Don't be fooled into thinking you're always straight up and sincere about every one of your actions and abilities. Remember the theory of cognitive dissonance in chapter 1? Humans are wily creatures. And while this certainly came into use thousands of years ago when we were hunting for food and shelter and figuring out ways not to be eaten by bloodthirsty predators, now we mostly use our cunning to find the quickest route to instant gratification while remaining as comfortable as possible.

DEPTH OF COMMITMENT

Steven Pressfield is one of my favorite authors. He wrote *Gates of Fire,* a fictional account of the Spartan Battle of Thermopylae, and the *The War of Art,* among many other brilliant books. In *Turning Pro,* his follow-up to *The War of Art,* he explains that the main difference between an amateur and a pro is their "depth of commitment. The amateur's commitment is shallow. The professional's is deep."

I love that concept of "being pro." Pros make the right choices; they commit and embrace adversity. They do the hard stuff. Amateurs accept being average. They show up when it's easy to show up and only then.

Pressfield believes depth of commitment can be developed and increased. We can move from shallow to deep. Often, deep commitment grows from the ashes of failure and shame, he says, which leads to self-respect. Pressfield makes his point with the story of his early years as a writer. He quit his job as a junior copywriter at an ad agency thinking that writing a novel would be an easy way to make a buck. Well, he never finished his first try. Seven years later, he says, "I'm dragging myself out of divorce, poverty, despair, blah blah, etc., thinking, 'Am I ready to try this same stunt again?'"

The difference this time around was Pressfield's depth of commitment. "This second time I am suitably chastened," he says. "I have had my butt handed to me and I know now how hard the job is and how much it is going to demand of me."

But this new novel flops and Pressfield says as a result his commitment grows deeper still. "In a way, failure is fuel for depth of commitment," he writes. "It raises the stakes. When our history is constituted entirely of Failure #1, Failure #2, and Failure #3, what else can we say to ourselves except, 'I will burst a blood vessel, I will pass out, will make my heart explode . . . but I will NOT crap out a fourth time!'"

The concept of "turning pro" means being brutally honest with yourself about how hard accomplishing something truly worthwhile is going to be, and being willing to give up a life that you've become very comfortable with in order to achieve it. Pressfield says it requires committing to conscious participation in the ongoing discovery of ourselves. He asks himself: "Is it a part-time gig? Or am I in it for keeps?"

We should ask the same question of ourselves. Commitment requires complete honesty. It means that you will do what you said you were going to do, even when you don't feel like doing it. Anything less is pointless. There's no "maybe" in commitment.

There's an expert ski run at Jackson Hole, Wyoming, called Corbet's Couloir that has been described as "America's scariest ski slope." To enter, a skier drops in from a cornice, a free fall of ten to twenty feet depending on snow conditions, that lands him or her in a narrow chute with jagged rock walls on either side. Once the skis leave the edge of that cornice, the skier is committed to threading that narrow couloir or getting real intimate with rock. Gravity doesn't allow for "maybe" or hesitation. The skier is all in.

That's exactly how a pro commits—upfront and clean with no hesitation or turning back. Educator and entrepreneur Peter Drucker said, "Unless commitment is made, there are only promises and hopes but no plans." By making a commitment to your True North, you step out of the role of interested observer and into the arena as active participant, where it's messy and scary and bloody.

So why don't we stop right here for a moment? Before your skis get ahead of you, I want you to be completely honest with yourself and those around you and answer this question: Will you commit to committing?

Excellent. Happy to hear it. Now, here's a little trick that'll make it easier to honor your promise to yourself: Make your commitment public. Tell somebody you respect. Tell a lot of people. A public commitment creates accountability. It's Psych 101, really: The desire to avoid embarrassment can be a powerful motivator. Studies show that making a public promise does work. Social psychologists Norbert Kerr and Robert MacCoun conducted one of the most telling studies that prove it. They wanted to investigate why some juries are unable to reach a verdict. Their conclusion revealed that hung juries are far more likely when jurors express their views in the presence of others, such as by a show of hands, instead of by secret ballot. Why? Pride. The researchers say that jurors who share their viewpoint publicly rarely change their position to avoid appearing weak-minded and indecisive.

Pride. Use it to your advantage. You can make public accountability even more effective by posting your commitment goals on social media and frequently updating your progress. Here's an example: In an experiment, researchers at Dominican University of California recruited 267 people from businesses, organizations, and networking groups for a study on goal achievement and accountability. The participants were randomly assigned to five groups:

Group 1 was asked to only think about business goals they wanted to accomplish in a four-week period and rank them by importance, and difficulty.

Groups 2 to 5 were given the same task but were instructed to actually write down their goals and rate them on paper.

Group 3 was also asked to write an action plan for each goal.

Group 4 also wrote an action plan but was asked to share their goals and action commitments with a friend.

Group 5 went the farthest by doing all of the above, but each also sent a detailed weekly progress report to a friend.

At the end of the study, the people who used more commitment tools achieved significantly more of their goals. Lead researcher Gail Matthews, PhD, reported that in Group 5, which publicly committed to their goals and shared weekly progress updates, 76 percent of participants either completed or nearly completed their goals. Compare that to just 43 percent of participants in Group 1, who only *thought* about their goals.

In the early days of Spartan Race, I found that a lot of people would sign up to compete and then just not turn up on the day. It was raining; their babysitter let them down; they were too tired after a week at the office and couldn't face the drive. The excuses were endless. I began to insist that those who wanted to participate had to organize coverage about it in their local paper or radio station. This was a way of getting them to be publicly accountable for their actions. It worked. Fall-off rates for races plummeted as participants were publicly on the hook for their commitment.

Consistency is not just a social norm, something we expect of others; commitment becomes an intrinsic part of our identity. Think of how a public commitment by President John F. Kennedy transformed the National Aeronautics & Space Administration (NASA). In 1962, NASA employees flicked on the television and heard the president declare to the world that the United States would put a man on the moon within eight years. Back then, NASA was just a small group of engineers and scientists with few of the technological resources to make Kennedy's promise a reality.

However, the president's statement turned a dream into an expectation with a deadline. It spurred pride and confidence in the men and women of NASA and supercharged their commitment to making history. And they did.

So how do you make your commitment public, and more important, how will you do it in a way that forces you to be accountable? You don't have to do an interview on local radio or national TV (though either would be good). You can simply look around and see who in your life is counting on you to commit to getting healthy, finding a job, building your business, freeing up your time, or doing whatever takes you toward your True North. Look around and see who will inspire you, believe in you, and root for you. They are the first people to share your commitment with.

Following that, you can take other steps to keep yourself on the hook. You can post your pledge on Facebook or tweet it on Twitter. You can tell your mailman or the woman who does your hair. The point is, get your purpose out there; make it real to you and others.

The other part of this strategy is to start narrowing your focus so that you can remain clear on exactly what it is you're working toward. When the Tendai-shu undertook *sennichi kaihōgyō,* their whole life centered on completing their goal. They only carried four items—a rope, a dagger, a book of maps of their route, and the different mantras to say at sacred locations. These items had an obvious practical purpose: They acted as a tangible motivation to bind themselves wholeheartedly to their goal. The monks never rested too long. Skipping a day of walking? Not a good decision. Doing so could both weaken their dedication and cause a crack in their commitment.

Don't allow your dedication to weaken either. Get rid of distractions. Focus on what's important, and learn to say "no" to anything that pulls you from the path of your commitments.

GET OFF THE COUCH!
How to Commit to Your Goal

Step I. WRITE DOWN YOUR PROMISE to yourself on an 8½ by 11 sheet of paper, sign it, date it, and tack it up somewhere like your bathroom mirror, where you will see it every day.

Here are some examples of promises you might make to yourself.

"I commit to . . ."

I commit to . . . do thirty burpees before breakfast every morning.

I commit to . . . leaving work by 6 p.m. every day and spending more time with my family.

I commit to . . . making five cold sales calls by phone before I move on to any other work.

I commit to . . . cutting processed foods out of my diet.

I commit to . . . saving an extra $100 a week for retirement.

I commit to . . . avoiding alcohol for thirty days.

I commit to . . . calling an old friend once a week and reestablishing long-dormant relationships.

I commit to . . . going to bed by 10 p.m. every night so I can be well rested for the next day.

I commit to . . . losing twenty-five pounds in the next thirty days.

I commit to . . . taking a continuing education course at a local college every semester to learn a new skill or broaden my base of knowledge.

I commit to . . . exercising for 30 minutes every day so I can prepare for a Spartan Race.

The simple act of writing down your promise to yourself in a contract-like document can go a long way toward motivating you to get moving. It's a physical sign—your first act of active engagement. You're not simply thinking about doing. You've started the showing up and doing part.

Step 2. CREATE A SOLID PLAN for active engagement that moves you toward your goal every day. See, talk is cheap, but that's what we humans do very well. Execution is hard. Always has been. Human beings procrastinate. They lack follow-through and self-control. The ancient philosophers Plato and Aristotle knew this and had a term for it, *akrasia,* a weak will. Willpower rarely ever works, and certainly not without definitive action. A plan for every day gives you the action that stokes your willpower. Think of it as your system for putting your contract into play. Systematic. Automatic. Routine. But powerful. It's like throwing lighter fluid on hot coals.

Commitment and preparation are critical for participation in a Spartan Race. That's why we offer the "Couch-to-Sprint Training Plan," a step-by-step exercise program that literally takes a sedentary couch spud from the cushions to standing at the starting line of a Spartan Sprint Race in just thirty-one days. If you commit to accomplishing each day's workout, your body and mind will be prepared for the challenge.

Set your plan in motion by answering these questions:
1. What will be different for me now that I've committed?
Sample answers:
I will wake up at 5 a.m. to write at least five hundred words of my memoir.

I will leave work early enough to be home in time to have dinner with my family every night.

I will stop watching sitcoms and get to bed by 10 p.m. every night.

If I watch TV, I will do twenty burpees or push-ups at every commercial break.

_____

_____

_____

_____

2. How will your work be different?

Sample answers:

I will have lunch or coffee with someone at my workplace that I don't know well once a week.

I will tackle my most challenging tasks during the three hours before lunch.

I will go for a run at lunchtime three days a week or do stretches in my office daily.

_____

_____

_____

_____

3. How will your relationships change?

Sample answers:

I will surround myself with people who share my values and goals and spend less time with people who don't support my goals.

I will spend more time with my kids and get to know their friends.

I will hand-write a letter to a friend I'm out of touch with or a letter of thanks to someone who has helped me in my life. One per week.

_____

_____

_____

_____

Action Tip: Put your active engagement plan in writing. Get yourself an old-school paper calendar, one that has lots of room on it to write, like those big desk calendars they sell at Staples. Every Sunday evening, map out your week. Write down the task, the act, the daily practice that will move you toward your weekly goals and, ultimately, your True North. There's something satisfying and motivating about crossing off that task when completed. Use a thick red grease pencil or a fat Sharpie. Don't be timid. When that task is done, relish in its completion with a satisfying mark, then move on to "next."

Step 3. MAKE IT PUBLIC. Ensure accountability by declaring your intentions to the world. Tweet your intended goal. Post it on your Facebook page. Tell your brother-in-law. Studies suggest you'll find it easier to be accountable to yourself by letting others know the commitment you're making to follow your True North. Make a list of key people with whom you will share your True North plan, and why?

Friends and family

Who_____

Why?_____

Who_____

Why?_____

Who_____

Why?_____

Supportive people you know professionally

Who_____

Why?_____

Who_____

Why?_____

Who_____

Why?_____

Step 4. FOLLOW A LEADER. Emulate someone whom you respect who has mastered commitment. A series of studies at the University of Georgia conducted a few years back suggests that self-control is contagious and hanging out with people who exhibit good self-control behavior—or even thinking about someone with strong self-control—can help you improve your own self-control.

> **TALK THE TALK**
> **I am seeking, I am striving, I am in it with all my heart.**
>
> —Vincent van Gogh

In one of the studies, the researchers assigned 112 volunteers to write about a friend with good self-control or a friend with bad self-control. On a later test of self-control (such as choosing whether or not to eat a cookie), those who wrote about friends with good self-control showed the greatest level of self-control.

Lead author Michelle vanDellen, writing in the journal *Personality and Social Psychology Bulletin,* explains that you don't have to share the same goal with someone to be influenced positively by their behavior. This influence crosses subject matters. For example, thinking about someone who demonstrates commitment by exercising regularly can make you more likely to stick to your career or financial goals or anything else that requires self-control on your part.

PRINCIPLE #3

FUEL YOUR ENTHUSIASM

Success is going from failure to failure without loss of enthusiasm.
—WINSTON CHURCHILL

People who never get carried away should be.
—MALCOLM FORBES

There's a spaghetti place in town. Good food, but the restaurant just wasn't doing well. I was there the other night and something had changed. They hired a new waiter. This guy was on the ball. He smiled. He was friendly and made us feel welcome. He was attentive and took charge when our order got mixed up. He made us laugh. We had the best time. I'm going back. Then it hit me: What was missing from this restaurant all these years was enthusiasm. This dude brought it in buckets.

Enthusiasm makes hard stuff easier. You could have a killer True North goal, but without enthusiasm your commitment is unlikely to last very long because hard things are rarely fun things. That's why passion is so friggin' valuable. I can almost guarantee that our waiter is going to turn that restaurant around. His enthusiasm was infectious to diners *and* other staff. In fact, I was thinking I should hire that waiter. I need to hire a social-media expert—you can teach web analytics, but you can't teach his brand of enthusiasm.

What you can do is be inspired by enthusiastic people, as I have been by the entrepreneur Elon Musk. Here's a guy, a visionary risk-taker, who made his first million at the age of twenty-eight with the sale of Zip2, a company he set up with his brother. He took the money and created another business, an online financial services company that eventually became PayPal. When eBay bought PayPal for $1.5 billion, Musk received $165 million and again reinvested much of that money into two new ventures, Space Exploration Technologies Corporation (SpaceX) and Tesla Motors. He's one of only two people in Silicon Valley to start three billion-dollar companies (the other guy being Jim Clark, who founded Silicon Graphics, Netscape, and WebMD). Musk's net worth is estimated at $19.1 billion, according to *Forbes*.

But money isn't really what Elon Musk is about. He is about financing his dreams and turning them into realities. Tesla's mission is to transport people to a carbon-free world with electric cars. SpaceX will someday relocate us to Mars. This is why he fascinates so many aspiring entrepreneurs: He's not a doer who dreams, he's a dreamer who does. "I don't create companies for the sake of creating companies," he says. "But to get things done."

That's a very Spartan attitude.

For all his astonishing triumphs, Musk's ride to billions hasn't been easy. He was raised in Pretoria, South Africa by a strict South African father and a British mother, who divorced when he was nine. Because he was small in stature and introverted by nature, he became a regular target for school bullies. On one occasion, his tormentors beat him so badly he had to be admitted to the hospital.

An interest in computers gave him a lifeline to hang on to. He received a Commodore VIC-20 at age nine and set about teaching himself programming. He was soon designing his own computer games. At the age of twelve, he even sold one for $500.

This ability to channel his focus into a passion even when the shit was hitting the fan in other areas of his life became a prominent factor in Musk's success, especially in 2008 when both Tesla and SpaceX fell deeply in debt. All of Musk's money, including the $165 million dollars he made from the sale of PayPal, had been invested into the businesses. Things weren't looking good. SpaceX was attempting a third launch of its rocket, the Falcon1. The previous two attempts had bombed. Launch day came. Bam. Another failure. The rocket plunged into the sea, losing all the satellites it had been contracted to carry for the Department of Defense and NASA.

Musk faced bankruptcy. He was in the middle of a divorce. Looking back on that time a few years later, he said, "I felt this is the closest I've ever come [to a nervous breakdown] because it seemed . . . pretty dark."

And yet, even as the darkness was closing in, he found the enthusiasm to move forward. His first step: Get out of bed. After that, put one foot in front of the other. He kept his ambition in focus and used it to build enthusiasm to push on in search of the financial support he needed. He found the money and planned another rocket launch; this time the rocket lifted off and made it into space. A few months later, NASA awarded SpaceX with the contract to transport US astronauts to the International Space Station. And a few months after that, Tesla raised $50 million in a venture capital round.

This wasn't luck. It was passion, perseverance, and enthusiasm in action.

THE SPIRIT WITHIN

"Enthusiasm" comes from the Greek word *entheos,* which means "the god, or spirit, within." It's the power inside us to pursue our highest dreams, to create and paint our extraordinary future, and face the most challenging of obstacles with optimism.

Enthusiasm is attractive. We want to be around people who are full of it. Courtney's enthusiasm for life is one of her most attractive traits. On our second date, she invited me to her apartment in Boston for an eggplant Parmesan dinner. Now, that's an ambitious move right there because I'm from an Italian family in Queens and I've had the best of the best eggplant Parm. I'm waiting in the living room and I can see her cooking away in the kitchen, frying those breaded eggplants. She turns and I see that she's wearing ski goggles and big gloves. "What the? Why are you in ski goggles?" I ask her. She answers, "So I won't get splattered by hot oil, obviously!"

Hey, okay, crazy lady. (She's Irish.) But I loved her enthusiasm.

I like to say enthusiasm is *energy giving.* It's opposite is apathy. Apathy is indifference, and laziness—which is *energy draining.* Stay away from people who are energy drainers. They will bring you down. And they're everywhere, even on a racecourse.

Recently, I ran a fifty-mile trail race with a buddy outside of Toronto. Canadians are normally very enthusiastic people, but there were a couple of volunteers on the course who were real curmudgeons. Not vocal. Not helpful. Downers. They didn't make the race any easier for me, and it was pretty tough already. I hadn't trained much for this race, so I wasn't quite ready for it. What's worse, it had rained for, like, ninety-eight days straight, so the trail was a muddy disaster. I wore these old smooth-bottom shoes that I love, instead of my new trail shoes. That was a big mistake.

I was slip-sliding and flopping on my face in this shit show. I was not in shape to run fifty miles and these two race volunteers were bringing me down. I realized that I had to do something to boost my enthusiasm or I was toast. So I started giving energy to everyone around me: "I might as well be wearing ice skates," I joked. "Hey, at least we're not running in Siberia!" I said any silly thing that came to mind to boost the mood.

Then, around mile twenty-eight, I started playing little mind games to keep myself up. I played this tape in my head: "If I can just get to thirty-two miles, I'll be okay. Then I know I can get to thirty-five miles and nudge myself to forty. Since, I've been running ten miles a day for weeks, I know I can handle the last ten, no problem."

You can build enthusiasm step by step. Once, I was out running ten miles with one of my sons and he didn't feel like going the distance. So I said, "Try this mental trick: Shake out your arms, now force yourself to smile a big stupid grin. Scientists have found that just by making the muscles in your face form a smile, you can make yourself instantly happy. Try it right now. See? Feel better?"

When people ask me how's my day, I say, "Awesome. How could my day be anything less? I'm alive, right? The sun's shining. The mountains are beautiful." You've got to love life. Don't be a fucking Grinch. Enthusiastic is much more appealing than miserable, isn't it?

The reason some people find enthusiasm so hard to sustain is that they haven't realized that it's nonnegotiable. Enthusiasm is the Spartan virtue of passion. Passion is what drives you to pursue a dream when the dream is all you have. It is the rocket fuel that blasts you past obstacles and over high hurdles. Without it, you'll sputter to a standstill when you are staggering under the weight of unthinkable challenges, and everyone is telling you that you're nuts. Trust me on this. I've been there. Many times.

3 BENEFITS OF FUELING YOUR ENTHUSIASM

1. You become more attractive to people. Think about the qualities in the people you love hanging out with. They are likely fun, energetic, action-oriented people who always seem to be up for anything. They exude enthusiasm, one of the most attractive of human qualities. Being enthusiastic, whether in a social or business setting, elevates the energy of the environment. It recruits the enthusiasm of others, and you become the sought-after leader that others want to be with.

2. You become more powerful and effective. It's hard to overstate the importance of body language, smiling, the tone of your voice when you are giving a speech. To be a powerful public speaker you need to engage your audience. You do that with enthusiasm. How many times have you listened to a boring speaker? He or she is timid, quiet, doesn't make eye contact, and speaks in a monotone. His body language transmits the message: "This isn't important; don't bother paying attention." A great speech needs to be larger than typical conversation. It requires more energy; it comes from your center. Remember the root of enthusiasm—"having God within"? It's the same with any performance or challenge, public or private: A larger-than-normal-life enthusiastic attitude empowers action and achievement.

3. You get things done. Enthusiasm is like a bellows that stokes a fire with oxygen. It's a heavy foot on a gas pedal. Enthusiasm is energy and urgency. You will accomplish more, do a better job, and have more fun in the process when you do what you're doing with enthusiasm. And when you're facing a setback or an obstacle, enthusiasm empowers the positive and you find the solution.

When I started Spartan Race, friends advised me not to finance another race project. The previous eight years had been a financial and psychological nightmare and now we were in the throes of one of the worst recessions in modern times. I had been battling to get Peak.com off the ground. I was obsessed with creating a race and community for extreme adventurers who, like me, wanted to be challenged to the max. But the interest was small-scale. There just weren't enough people out there at the time chomping at the bit to be tested to the extreme—both physically and mentally. Instead I was hauling ass over hot coals in business, and getting severely burned in the process. I had spent two million dollars and was completely over-leveraged. When I started talking to friends and family about Spartan they looked at me like I had lost my mind. Maybe I had. But the idea wouldn't go away. I kept thinking: "What if I pulled back a bit?" Changed the race from a week in the wilderness to a three- or five-hour event? Made it more accessible to all types of people whose lives needed the kind of testing conditions of an extreme physical challenge? I realized then that the brutal terrain of Peak.com was a pathway leading me to Spartan. Of course, building this new company was not going to be easy. I would have to finance it myself through what little savings I had and by maxing out credit cards. I had burned a lot of financial bridges with Peak investors who may have been interested but were facing their own towering problems now. The world was in a severe economic shakeout. It was the worst time to be setting up a business.

But I had ambition and enthusiasm. And, well, not much of anything else, but those two things fueled my motivation. My ambition was to create an extreme sporting event for the masses to get people off the couch; my enthusiasm was the hunger I had, after my experience with Peak, to make it a success. Knowing I could not live with another failure was what got me out of bed every morning and through the darkest nights of the soul that came with building Spartan.

Over the years, I've come to understand that motivation involves three factors that have to work in unison:

Activation is the decision to start. You activated your new journey when you committed to pursuing your True North.

Persistence is the continued effort toward a goal even though obstacles may exist. I have a goal of doing three hundred burpees every morning. Sometimes I don't feel like doing them, so I make a decision to start and then ten turns into twenty. Twenty turns into fifty, and so on. As long as I persist, I will finally reach my goal.

Intensity is the focus and energy that goes into pursuing a goal.

INCENTIVIZING ACTION

There are a number of interesting theories about what spurs people to act. Most of the research is about extrinsic or intrinsic motivation. Extrinsic motivation is driven by external rewards such as money, fame, trophies, and recognition, while intrinsic motivation is stimulated from within by deep-rooted values, satisfaction, or joy.

If you were to ask a lot of people whether they'd like cold hard cash as a reward for running their first marathon or whether the innate sense of accomplishment would be reward enough, most wouldn't hesitate to say, "Show me the money!" However, studies have shown that external rewards like money, while awesome in the moment, don't keep you motivated to continue for the long term. Daniel Pink is an expert in this area. He says that extrinsic motivation can quickly promote bad behavior, create addiction, and encourage short-term thinking at the expense of the long view.

HOW TO FIND THE ENTHUSIASM TO GET IN SHAPE

Need some scientific motivation to lace up your running shoes at 5 a.m.?

How does turning back your biological clock nine years sound? Honestly, I haven't needed to find motivation to exercise in forty years. Working out makes me feel great and I couldn't live without my morning routine. But then I read about this study out of Brigham Young University. This is the gravy: After analyzing data from more than 5,800 Americans, exercise scientists at BYU figured out that people who are highly physically active are actually biologically younger than their chronological age by almost ten years. They discovered this by measuring these things at the ends of our chromosomes called telomeres. Telomeres are like those plastic nubs on the ends of your shoelaces that keep them from unraveling. Apparently, they are a highly accurate measure of cellular aging. The older you become, the shorter your telomeres. But the researchers found that women who jogged for at least thirty minutes a day and men who ran at least 40 minutes daily had longer telomeres. The highly active folks were seven years more biologically youthful than people who were moderately active and nine years younger than inactive adults. Imagine: You could be physically younger than your birth certificate declares! How's that as incentive for another round of burpees?

Think about it: If you're only doing a job that you hate because the money is good, you may be able to afford a new car but you'll be miserable driving it. If you're only going to the gym because you want to lose weight, not because you enjoy it, I guarantee you'll soon stop going. External rewards are fleeting.

Intrinsic motivation, on the other hand, keeps the fire stoked. Here's scientific proof: Back in the early 1970s, a group of psychologists conducted an experiment with preschool kids who loved to draw. Some of the children were given crayons and paper and told to have fun. A second group was told that if they drew a picture, they would receive a cool "good player" certificate, complete with silky ribbon. A couple of weeks later, the same activity was introduced back into the class. This time the scientists found that the kids who drew in order to win the ribbon (the extrinsic reward) showed much less intrinsic interest in drawing than those who had taken part purely for the enjoyment of drawing.

So which kid do you want to be? The one with a silky ribbon or the one who draws simply for the enjoyment it brings?

THE MINDSET TEST

Stanford University psychologist Carol Dweck says how you acknowledge success plays a key role in creating intrinsic motivation. Dweck has spent decades examining why some people are motivated to achieve more than others and defines her research within the simple but powerful idea that people have one of two mindsets. Those with a "fixed mindset" assume that character, intelligence, talent, and abilities are as rigid as a rock and cannot be changed; and success will come to those blessed with the right smarts, skills, and strengths. People with a "growth mindset" believe that

BEWARE OF THE ENTHUSIASM KILLER

When you experience multiple setbacks, it's human nature to see yourself as a victim, which is about the worst thing you can do in a tough situation. Fight that feeling. Nothing crushes enthusiasm like throw-up-your-hands self-pity and catastrophizing. Psychologists have a name for these enthusiasm killers: ANTS, *Automatic Negative Thoughts.* Thinking to yourself, "I'll never get this venture off the ground because I'll never raise the startup capital," can be a self-fulfilling prophecy. Complaining that there's nothing you can do to lose your gut because you've been cursed with a slow metabolism, is not only a major buzz kill, it'll guarantee failure before you even start. Bruce Lee once said, "As you think, so shall you become." Remember this the next time ANTS start crawling inside your head.

talents and capabilities can be developed, and they see failure not as evidence of incompetence or weakness, but as a challenge to themselves to stretch and improve. Most of us adopt one of these two mindsets when we are children. From then on we apply "fixed" or "growth" thinking to our daily behaviors, which colors our relationship with success and failure.

As part of her investigation into this topic, Dweck carried out a study with 128 fifth-graders. The students were separated into groups and given a simple IQ test. One group was told it performed really well and was praised *for being smart.* The other group was told it performed really well and was praised *for effort.* The researchers then asked the kids if they wanted to take another easy test or opt for a harder one. The majority of those kids praised for their intelligence jumped on the easy option, while 90 percent of those praised for their hard work were up for the more difficult challenge. Why? Dweck says the "smart kids" didn't want to appear stupid so they decided to hedge their bets by doing an easier quiz. The praise they were given told them they had an innate intelligence and they wanted to protect this view of themselves. The children who were praised for their effort, however, reasoned that if they put in even more effort, there was a good chance they might achieve better results. They saw themselves as being in control of their success, while the others, who were told their intelligence was fixed, saw themselves as having no control over their success.

Henry Ford once said, "Whether you think you can or whether you think you can't, you're right," and the premise here is more or less the same. If you enthusiastically believe in your ability to succeed, you are more likely to persevere with passion and reach your goal.

GET OFF THE COUCH!
How to Stoke Your Enthusiasm

Step 1. MAKE YOUR GOAL WORTHY OF YOUR ENTHUSIASM. For decades, organizational psychologists Gary Latham and Edwin Locke have analyzed more than one thousand studies on motivation and task performance for their research on goal setting. They found that simply telling yourself to "do your best" is ineffective for reaching your goal. Ninety percent of the time, having a special goal that could be measured (such as beating your last 10K time or doing ten more burpees today than you did last week) and was difficult led to better performance than easier, less specific goals. If the challenge isn't difficult enough to seem significant to you, they argue, how could that motivate you to work harder? Enthusiasm is fueled by significant challenge and the reward of feeling great once the goal is achieved.

Another way to define "significant challenge" is "ambition," and ambition is different from motivation. Ambition is the desire to accomplish something you believe would be amazing. Motivation is the reason for behaving in a specific way to achieve a goal. They are different, but you cannot be successful without having both, as the chart below illustrates.

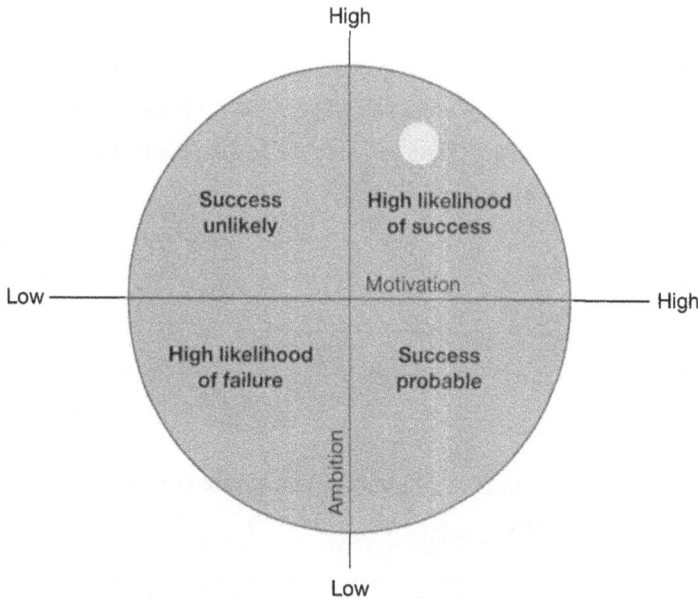

Step 2. EVALUATE YOUR MOTIVATION. Use the graph to map today's motivation and ambition. Write a brief description of what is going on in your life today that impacts your motivation and what you are trying to accomplish.

Today:

On a scale of 1 to 10, 10 being very high, rate your level of motivation today:

_____

On a scale of 1 to 10, 10 being very high, rate your level of ambition today:

_____

Considering your ratings, describe your likelihood of success:

_____

Use the graph to map your future motivation and ambition. Write a brief description of what you hope to accomplish in the future. Also include what's going on in your life that is impacting your level of motivation for your goal.

Future:

_____

_____

_____

On a scale of 1 to 10, 10 being very high, rate your level of motivation today:

_____

On a scale of 1 to 10, 10 being very high, rate your level of future ambition:

_____

Considering your ratings, describe your likelihood of success:

_____

Do this exercise several times as you work toward your goal.

What patterns did you notice when you were successful?

_____

_____

_____

What patterns did you notice when you were NOT successful?

_____

_____

_____

What changes will you have to make to improve your likelihood of success?

_____

_____

_____

Step 3. BOOST ENTHUSIASM WITH A GSD PLANNER THAT HELPS YOU RECOGNIZE "LITTLE WINS." GSD stands for Get Shit Done! Planner. Its purpose is to:
* Map out the goals to your True North.
* Identify small steps and keep them firmly in mind.
* Track and celebrate little wins.
* Keep you motivated, ambitious, and honest.

Devise your own personalized Get Shit Done! Planner on your computer, phone, or in a notebook. Or use the five-week (thirty-six-day) sample GSD Planner in the appendix. See an example on page 69.

HOW TO BUILD ENTHUSIASM
Science-based tricks for
summoning zest

Fake it. You can fire up your enthusiasm simply by *acting* enthusiastic. Harvard Business School researchers figured this one out in the famous "power pose" study. In the experiment, forty-two men and women were randomly divided into "high" or "low" power pose groups. Both groups gave saliva samples before posing to measure levels of the stress hormone cortisol and the power hormone testosterone. Then participants were instructed to strike either a slouching, diminutive pose, or a powerful pose occupying more space with feet spread strongly, chest out, hands on hips. The subjects were asked to maintain these poses for five minutes while preparing for a job interview. As expected, the high-power posers reported feeling significantly more powerful than the low-power posers before the interview. And follow-up saliva tests showed greater levels of the dominance hormone testosterone and less cortisol, the exact opposite of the levels found in the low-power posers. Now, if striking a superhero pose before your next job interview or at the starting line of your next triathlon just isn't going to happen, try something more natural and palatable: smiling or taking a brisk walk before an important meeting, using positive imagery, or doing ten burpees before a race. Thinking positive thoughts or moving your body triggers the release of endorphins that promote positive feelings, says Hendrie Weisinger, PhD, author of *Performing Under Pressure: The Science of Doing Your Best When It Matters Most*. Watch any athlete or team during warm-ups. They typically do a brisk walk-through, both physically and mentally, that primes the pump of enthusiasm before the contest.

Talk to yourself in the third person. Studies by researchers at the University of Michigan and University of California at Berkeley suggest that positive self-talk can drive enthusiasm more effectively during stressful situations when people refer to themselves using second-person pronouns such as "you," *You can make this shot!* Or by using your name. *Lisa, just keep moving your feet! Sara, you can do it!* In the study, participants who avoided first-person pronouns, like I and me, were calmer and more confident and they performed tasks better. The researchers believe that the subtle shift in language can help people better focus their thoughts and manage their feelings during performance stress.

Get fired up. In the film *Hoosiers,* Gene Hackman plays the coach of a small Indiana high school basketball team that defies the odds to win the state championship in 1952. Before each game, he gathers his team in a huddle and starts them clapping louder and faster with increasing enthusiasm before they take the court. The tactic replaces feelings of fear that can overwhelm and distract us from doing our best with the fuel of success—enthusiasm. Try a little clapping therapy to goose up your enthusiasm for whatever task is before you.

Crank it up. "Roar," "Don't Stop Believin'," "Fight Song," Jimi Hendrix's "Purple Haze," whatever rocks your world, that is. Music is a powerful motivator and many studies have proven it can improve performance, athletic or otherwise. When listening to music you love, your brain releases the pleasure-inducing chemical dopamine, which counteracts cortisol and distracts from fatigue. Sports psychologist Dr. Costas Karageorghis of Brunel University in London likens music to "a type of legal performance-enhancing drug." Music can increase endurance by keeping people awash in strong emotions, especially if the athlete identifies strongly with the emotions in the song.

Visualize yourself finishing the race or endeavor. Visualization has been a time-honored tactic for reducing pre-competition jitters and improving performance since Soviet Olympic athletes started using it in the 1970s. Now, almost every successful athlete uses some version of visualization, for example, walking through an entire round of golf, a tennis match, or other performance while engaging his or her senses in a mental rehearsal. Brain studies show that mental imagery impacts the same processes as actually performing the physical act, from motor control to concentration. Visualization can even enhance motivation. Sports legends like Tiger Woods and Jack Nicklaus, and NBA greats Jerry West and Michael Jordan, have all attributed making game-winning shots to rehearsing making those same shots countless times in their mind's eye. Get in the practice of visualizing your big shots, finishing the race, writing the book, completing the report, losing the pounds, turning a profit. Each time before preparing to tackle a challenge, take thirty seconds, close your eyes, and visualize your success. See if it makes a difference in your enthusiasm or performance.

To test the psych-you-up power of visualization, scientists reporting recently in the *Journal of Strength and Conditioning Research* recruited sixteen sprinters and ran them through a battery of timed sprints. In one part of the experiment, the sprinters were asked to close their eyes for thirty seconds and visualize themselves setting a sprint personal-best record prior to a run of thirty meters. In the control experiment, the sprinters were instructed to count backwards from one thousand by sevens for thirty seconds prior to the same run, which effectively distracted them from thinking about the upcoming sprint. The researchers found that the sprinters' performance improved significantly after the visualization exercise compared to after the distraction experiment. The greatest difference occurred during the acceleration phase—the first ten meters of the race. Here's something more to think about. The greatest improvement occurred when sprinters ran the timed interval within two minutes of the psych-up. The benefit virtually vanished if the runners waited three or five minutes after completing the visualization before racing.

HEY (YOUR NAME HERE) GET SHIT DONE!

MY TRUE NORTH:	
For the week of:	
Big Idea Goal: (Ambition) Linked to your True North	
This week's goal: (Motivation)	
This week's Small Steps:	
Monday	
Tuesday	
Wednesday	

The Spartan Way

Thursday	
Friday	
Saturday	
Sunday	
This week's Little Wins:	
Monday	
Tuesday	
Wednesday	
Thursday	
Friday	
Saturday	
Sunday	
How do you feel?	

PRINCIPLE #4

DELAY GRATIFICATION

In reading the lives of great men, I found that the first victory they won was

over themselves . . . self-discipline with all of them came first.

—HARRY S. TRUMAN

Self-control is like a muscle; the more you exercise it the stronger it gets. Every time you avoid something that tempts you, you strengthen your resolve to resist future temptations. This is an important principle to understand because it's such a powerful tool for success. In almost any area in which you want to achieve something worthwhile—in your career, relationships, finances, or health—one of the most effective personality traits is being able to delay gratification.

I started practicing this at a very young age—I'd say, before I turned ten. I remember turning off our car's air conditioning and rolling up the windows in the summertime to see how long I could take the discomfort and delay the blast of cold air. In the wintertime, believe it or not, I'd take cold showers (still do to this day). I'd even carry rocks around the neighborhood to toughen up. I think hearing my mother talk about the discipline of yoga and meditation gave me these strange ideas. She used to go to meditation camps where participants would sit for days pondering an unanswerable question. I remember her telling me it how difficult but enlightening it was.

Delaying gratification is a heavy dumbbell to lift, and it helps to understand why. Self-control takes significant effort because we are hard-wired to seek pleasure. Pleasure motivates us to act. It's how we survived. By controlling your behavior you learn the potential future rewards of delaying pleasure.

A famous experiment in 1960 explored the benefits of delaying gratification. Maybe you've heard about the marshmallow test devised by Stanford University professor Walter Mischel. In the study, he gave nursery-school kids a choice: They could eat a marshmallow now or wait awhile and get two marshmallows to eat. It turned out that only one in three children chose to wait for the second treat. The rest went for instant gratification.

For the next thirty years, these same kids were watched as they grew from toddlers to teens to adults. That's where the really interesting findings bubbled up. The kids who were able to hold out for the second marshmallow tended to get better grades in school and turn into healthier adults. They had good jobs and successful relationships. When the kids who couldn't delay gratification became adults, Mischel noticed that a greater percentage of them were obese, school dropouts, or had drug problems. Some had even served prison time.

The general results of the test weren't necessarily a revelation. After all, patience is a virtue that has been celebrated by many down through the ages. The Spartans honored patience. They trained their warriors for up to ten years before they went into battle. And the writer, philosopher, and one of America's Founding Fathers Benjamin Franklin correctly pointed out, "He that can have patience can have what he will." But the specific outcomes did get scientists and educators wondering whether the kids who could delay their gratification had a natural capacity for endurance and, as a consequence, for success, or whether patience was a trait that could be learned.

Over the last few decades, other researchers mimicked Mischel's test and got similar results. I tried Mischel's "marshmallow test" on my son Jack when he was six years old. I told him he could have one scoop of ice cream instantly or two scoops if he waited fifteen minutes. He thought about it a little, then asked, "How long will I have to wait for fifteen scoops?" Already, my kid had figured out that greater things can come to those who wait.

Delaying gratification is like catching lightning in a bottle. It's hard to do, especially when you're struggling with money. When I started Spartan, I said we would stand on certain principles and never bend under pressure. We would not align ourselves with partners who we felt would pull us down. My investors went crazy when we turned down a lot of potential partners—like Red Bull. I just wouldn't do it. I said I'm just not feeding people poison. So we left a lot of money on the table for fifteen years. But I learned from my mistakes. If you burn your hand on the stove, you quickly figure out that you should never put your hand there again.

Patience eventually becomes power. When you are a master of your choices, you are not a slave to impulses, bad habits, and the whims of other people. When you couple delayed gratification with perseverance, you have a commanding weapon in your utility belt, which is why it's a core Spartan virtue.

Clearly, it's easier said than done. Most people have trouble with the idea of delaying gratification. The thinking is, why deny yourself anything when it's all so easy to get? Why go without speedy internet connection, 24/7 social media, same-day deliveries, hookups online, movies on demand, fast food, easy credit, and everything else that can come at the push of a button? If it's all there, then why not engage?

The fact is, by buying into instant gratification, you're buying into ineptitude. A life where everything is done for you at the click of a mouse does not prepare you to deal with life's real complexities. Just think about how out of touch you felt when you lost your cell phone. You grew anxious. Who couldn't reach you? What "urgent" messages were you missing? Think about the last time your house lost power in a storm and you had to go without a computer, television, and the internet for a few hours or days. Compare that inconvenience with a real problem like illness, loss of job, marriage breakdown, caring for aging parents, or getting help for teenagers on drugs. How will you manage real crises like those when you struggle without an Internet connection for a few days?

I found this study interesting: Ramesh Sitaraman, a computer science professor at the University of Massachusetts at Amherst, studied 6.7 million internet users to see how long most were willing to wait for a page or video to load. He found that most people waited two seconds before impatience got the better of them. After five seconds, 25 percent of users had moved on. In another study conducted for the Pew Research Center in Washington, D.C., experts concluded that young people's thirst for instant gratification by being constantly connected to the internet forces them to make "quick, shallow choices." It makes sense: How can you make an informed decision if you're only giving yourself two seconds to make it?

Don't blame Al Gore. The problem of instant gratification was not spawned by the creation of the internet. It's not a modern phenomenon. It has an evolutionary backstory. Our cavemen ancestors were hard-wired to hunt smaller, easier-to-catch prey rather than delay eating in hopes that a large animal would stroll by and provide them with a week's worth of hearty meals. We've carried that urgency in our genetic code through the ages, but now our urgent needs include Starbucks Iced Coconut Milk Mocha Macchiato and the latest iPhone.

For a lot of people, the big problem with delayed gratification is that the pay-off is gradual and subtle. It doesn't arrive in a box with a bow and a band playing behind it. For example, you are healthier after you've vanquished your sugar addiction or your smoking habit. But you can't really see the difference. You still look a lot like you did before quitting.

Pay-offs usually emerge slowly and not very dramatically. So it helps to recognize that delaying gratification is not just a means to an end. It's a tool. Those kids who resisted the marshmallow in Mischel's test didn't know that they were laying the foundation stone of a remarkable inner strength. You're doing the same thing. The more you practice delaying gratification, the easier it will become. Just as lifting weights regularly strengthens muscles, exerting willpower at regular intervals toughens disciple and strengthens resolve. Now, combine some of that weight lifting with willpower practice, and you may see your self-discipline soar. Get this: Researchers at Macquarie University in Sydney, Australia, found that people who practiced self-discipline along with getting regular physical exercise actually became more disciplined in ALL areas of their lives.

HIT THE PAUSE BUTTON

My friend Zach Even-Esh, the founder of The Underground Strength Gym, is one of the most disciplined people I know. He is a tough guy who had a tough life. He was a wrestler, a body builder, one strong dude, but he suffered from debilitating depression for years. Then, one day he woke up and announced to himself: "That's enough, I'm done being depressed.

WHAT I'VE LEARNED
Mark Divine, former Navy SEAL, CEO of SEALFIT, and author of UNBEATABLE MIND

Discipline is about managing your emotions. [Emotional] stress is just resistance. We can't eradicate stress in our lives. We are hard-wired to respond to it. The key is to change your relationship with stress so that when you approach that resistance, you embrace it. You embrace the suck. You look at that resistance and say, "That is going to make me strong. You are my teacher." You create a new relationship to that stress.

I'm never going to allow myself to go back to this feeling of merely existing. I want to live. Today is gonna be a beautiful day!" That moment changed him forever, and he never looked back.

Zach changed his thought patterns and defeated his inner demons by training like a man possessed—two long sessions a day, running and rucking, hitting bodyweight circuits as soon as he woke up; then training on the beach, in the woods, in his garage, at his gym. Anywhere and everywhere. He worked out with Navy SEALs and completed their brutal program called the 20X challenge. "Not once did the thought of *quit* ever creep into my mind," he says.

Zach credits his transformation to delaying gratification. And the key step to mastering that skill is what he calls "knowing your *why.*" Knowing your why is the same thing as knowing your True North. It's your purpose and passion for living. When you know your why, delaying gratification becomes easier. Your choices become more meaningful because you know why you are making them. They are relevant to your very core.

Not long after completing the 20X challenge, Zach faced another extreme: Hurricane Sandy hit his hometown. The East Coast superstorm destroyed homes. It destroyed lives. It challenged the survival of Zach's own business. But knowing his *why* "allowed me to be strong in mind, body, and spirit for my family while stress was all around me," Zach says.

Zach also lives his life according to another principle, a quote by entrepreneur Jim Rohn: "We must all suffer from one of two pains: The pain of discipline and the pain of regret. The difference is discipline weighs ounces while regret weighs tons."

MAKE A PLAN

No one wakes up ready-loaded with self-discipline after a lifetime of being led by his or her impulses. You need a plan. You have to strategize. Remember, principles are just words without a series of actions, and that's what a plan delivers.

One requirement of achieving the Spartan way of life is changing eating habits from calorie-dense to nutrient-rich. This means eating lots of whole foods—food that is as close to its natural form as possible, like fruits, vegetables, beans and legumes, nuts, grass-fed meats, seafood, and eggs. However, if you've been filling your fridge—and your body—with processed snack foods and fast-food meals for the last few decades, going cold turkey on Kentucky Fried Chicken may be hard to do. You may need to wean yourself off the deep-fried and packaged Frankenfoods. How? Start slowly but deliberately. Plan to cut back on added sugars. Start with gradually using less sugar and half-and-half in your morning coffee until you love drinking it black. Cut one meal of burgers, fries, or pizza out of your weekly menu. Then, slowly replace those meals with healthier fare

WHAT SPARTANS EAT

Whole foods. Fill up on with fresh fruits, vegetables, beans and legumes, lean grass-fed meats, seafood, and eggs.

Limited processed foods. Avoid stuff in boxes and cans, foods that can last in your pantry for weeks. They are filled with preservatives, sodium, and trans fats. They will kill you.

Nothing. Sometimes Spartans fast to keep ourselves honest and gritty and feeling alive. Try skipping dinner occasionally.

Only when we're hungry. Spartans don't snack.

The best of what's available and needed. In other words, Spartans adapt their diets to the seasons, eating what's fresh and locally grown, if possible. The closer to home you find whole foods, the more nutritious they tend to be.

until you can limit indulging in burgers to once every two weeks, then no more than once a month. You can still have a burger now and then; you're just learning to delay gratification. And I guarantee you'll enjoy that cheeseburger that much more when you do indulge.

Building up your delayed-gratification muscles can have a big impact on your health. Check this out: A recent report in the journal *Preventive Medicine* linked delaying immediate gratification with fewer visits to fast-food restaurants. Restaurant food is typically energy-dense and nutrient-poor. Knowing that food consumed away from home increases one's risk for obesity and other chronic illnesses, researchers were curious if this could be linked to economic behavior. So they organized a study. A team

WHAT I'VE LEARNED

When (money) becomes the sole goal, there are sacrifices. I still
drive the broken-down 2004 used Volkswagen Golf I always have.
I've found that the low-burn lifestyle as opposed to ever more
money gives you an incredible amount of leverage because, in
the worst-case scenario, you're covered.

—Tim Ferriss, author, entrepreneur

of scientists from the American Cancer Society and several universities analyzed responses from 5,871 US adults who took a survey about lifestyle habits, including fast-food eating. The subjects were asked whether they would prefer to receive $10 immediately or a larger sum ($12, $15, or $18) in thirty days. Results clearly showed a correlation between the willingness to wait for more cash and fewer bacon cheeseburgers and curly fries eaten. Study participants who most often chose the delayed dollar amount were 26 percent less likely to eat fast-food than those who chose to get the cold hard cash right away.

Here's an idea: If you want to lose twenty pounds before your next Spartan Race, give a buddy a hundred bucks and tell him or her to donate it to charity if you can't meet your goal.

Money certainly motivates people. But so do little steps that produce little wins that spur you on to create big changes. Getting back to weaning off added sugar. Little by little, in time, you'll find that your cravings for sweets will cease and your palate will change. Coffee black will be delicious and you won't need the coffee cake to go with it. Wean yourself off restaurant foods and eventually you will find them way too salty for your taste buds. The next fast-food burrito you'll eat will make you physically sick from all the sodium. You'll find baked goods, candy, and ice cream will change for you as well. Candy will be too sweet and you'll prefer a piece of whole fruit for dessert. You'll be drinking water rather than soda, and you won't miss the carbonated crap at all. Trust me, this happens. Eating regularly and healthily to maintain stable blood-sugar levels will help to strengthen your willpower.

HOW EATING SUGAR MAKES DELAYING GRATIFICATION HARDER

Americans consume roughly thirty-two teaspoons of added sugars every day. That's according to the U.S. Department of Agriculture. That's a real pile of trouble. Many medical experts say sugar in our diets may be the most significant health threat in America. In fact a 2014 editorial in *JAMA Internal Medicine* announced: "Too much sugar does not just make us fat; it can also make us sick."

The reason sugar is such a troublemaker is how it messes with our bodies and makes it harder to say "no" to more sugar in the future. Like a drug, it tickles the pleasure center in our brains and causes us to want more and more. Eating sugar retrains your taste buds, causing you to require more and more sugar to enjoy the same sweetness. And when you're eating more sugar, you're eating less healthy food the rest of the day. An analysis of dozens of studies in *Nutrition Research* found a distinct association between higher added sugar intake and poorer diet and lower intake of important nutrients. That's because of the way sugar works in your body. Say you drink a glass of "fruit juice" made with *high fructose corn syrup* (HFCS), a man-made sweetener. Immediately, the sugar rush in your blood causes your body to flood your system with insulin to deal with the toxic overload. But that influx of insulin can yank too much sugar out of the bloodstream, causing an energy crash. And that affects your brain. When your brain runs low on glucose (sugar), you become foggy, less attentive, more irrational, making you less likely to be able to control your impulses. And you go hunting urgently for another quick sugar dose. The vicious cycle continues over and over. That's how sugar can destroy your best dietary intentions. It blows the willpower out of your brain.

And that's not the worst of it. When you regularly cycle through blood glucose swings, your insulin becomes less effective at its job of shuttling excess sugar out of the bloodstream. This is known as insulin resistance, and it's the precursor to a terrible and terribly common disease known as type 2 diabetes. Heart disease is another symptom of living the sweet life. People who get 25 percent or more of their calories from added sugar are more than twice as likely to die from heart disease as those who eat less than 10 percent. The brain suffers from a sugar addiction, too. Recent studies have linked high blood sugar to both depression and dementia. In a study in the journal *Diabetologica,* researchers found that high blood sugar lowers levels of a neurochemical called *brain-derived neurotropic factor* (BDNF) that helps brain cells communicate, build memories, learn new tasks, and, it's safe to add, bolster your willpower to delay gratification.

BE DELIBERATE

It's also necessary to get real about your current behaviors. If your goal is to start training, stop smoking, or build a business, what habits and actions have been holding you back? As Chinese military strategist and philosopher Sun Tzu wrote, "If you know neither the enemy nor yourself, you will succumb in every battle." Once you know the enemy, say *"no"* to it. Can't do that? Well, then start with a *"not now."* That's a step in the right direction and similar to the strategy above. It helps you to be less hasty and more deliberate in your decision-making. You are building mental strength. These two small words can give you a moment's pause to rethink your action every time you consider blowing off a run or lighting up a cigarette. It provides just enough time for your rational brain to overcome your impulse for instant gratification. Continuous *not nows* will eventually lead you to your emphatic *no.*

DEALING WITH SETBACKS

You may feel that your efforts just aren't cutting it. You still have cravings. You don't love getting up at 5 a.m. for a workout; in fact, you'd rather be in bed. That's okay. Kelly McGonigal, a psychologist who teaches a class on the science of willpower at Stanford, says self-control is about holding two opposite options in your mind. The first is the knowledge that you control the choice to pick one or the other. And the second is that you can choose instant gratification or the action that's best for you. Hell, most of us would like to turn over for a longer snooze when the alarm goes off at 5 a.m. The truth is, you won't. If you've created a powerful enough *why,* you'll choose to get up because, very simply, you know it is up to you. Only you can do it.

Finally, eliminate temptations and distractions from your environment. This isn't rocket science. It's just smart behavior. If you want to create better eating habits, don't leave junk food in your kitchen. If you want to focus on following your True North, eliminate the clutter in your home and simplify your life to reduce the unimportant things that compete for your time. If you're trying to kick a bad cell phone habit, switch it off and put it in a drawer when you are at home. In Walter Mischel's test, the kids who couldn't keep their eyes off the marshmallow were less likely to resist it than were the children who closed their eyes or turned away. "We've found a way to really improve human choice and freedom," Mischel, now eighty-eight, told *The New Yorker* recently. "If we have the skills to allow us to make discriminations about when we do or don't do something, when we do or don't drink something, and when we do and when we don't wait for something, we are no longer victims of our desires."

Managing your impulses is also the Spartan Way to push upward in life, to break through those barriers that have been holding you back. Learning through practice is how it happens. Practice turning off the TV. Practice saying "no" to dessert. Stop eating the foods you shouldn't be eating. Start doing the exercise you should be doing. Put down your tablet or your smart phone, at least for a few hours a day. Get up early. Take cold showers. Strengthen discipline by practicing discipline. People make excuses. I've heard them all. You have, too. Or else you're the one making them. Don't be. Most excuses are bullshit.

Be ruled or rule. That's what it comes down to.

GET OFF THE COUCH!
How to Learn to Delay Gratification

Step 1. TURN DOWN THE HEAT. When you want something immediately, you're like a defensive end chasing a quarterback. You're
in hot pursuit, out for blood, drooling for the taste of quarterback
sack. One way to temper that urgent desire is to mentally cool
down. Get out of that hot environment. If your future goal is to
fit into your tuxedo for your kid's wedding and you find yourself
staring at a triple scoop of Ben & Jerry's, walk out of the ice-cream
shop. Literally put distance between yourself and the object of
instant gratification. You've heard the phrase, out of sight, out of
mind? Add *out of mouth* and you have one of the best mantras for
cutting processed foods out of your diet. Do this: Grab a heavy-
duty garbage bag and go through your fridge and pantry. Throw
out the candy, cookies, crackers, soft drinks—any carb-heavy,
chemical-laden packaged foods. Don't replace them. If they aren't
in your home, you can't eat them.

Step 2. MAKE IT UGLY. Change your perception of an appealing
object or action you wish to resist. Want a third cocktail? Think of
the last time you puked in the bushes from too much tequila.
One of the kids in Mischel's experiment pictured a frame around
his marshmallows to make the temptation less immediate and
harder to get to. In his book *The Marshmallow Test: Mastering
Self-Control,* Mischel describes how he used visualization to help
him quit his cigarette habit in the 1960s. Each time he craved a
cigarette, he created a picture in his mind of a lung-cancer patient
hunched over and decrepit with a shaved head. He saw that as his
potential future. When he did, he reframed the appeal of the instant gratification of a smoke. He has been smoke-free ever since.

Step 3. MAKE YOUR GOAL THE GRATIFICATION. Self-control simply comes down to contemplating the choice between two options and always choosing the one with the grander reward that aligns with your True North. You can use what you've learned about delaying gratification from Mischel's marshmallow test in combination with the powerful technique of taking small steps to help you make the right choices. Use this exercise to start saying "not now" to the marshmallows in your life.

Spot Your Marshmallows

Identify your sweetest marshmallows at home, at work, in your relationships, and your health. Recognize and record how these immediate rewards will knock you off your path away from your True North.

MARSHMALLOWS AT HOME

MARSHMALLOW IDENTIFIED	HOW THIS TAKES ME AWAY FROM MY TRUE NORTH	SMALL STEP I CAN TAKE TO SAY "NOT NOW"
1.Example: Facebook	Spending 3 hours a night on Facebook takes me away from spending time with my family.	At the end of the day I will give myself half an hour before I go to bed to check Facebook.
2.		
3.		

MARSHMALLOWS AT WORK

MARSHMALLOW IDENTIFIED	HOW THIS TAKES ME AWAY FROM MY TRUE NORTH	SMALL STEP I CAN TAKE TO SAY "NOT NOW"
1. Example: Going out for a drink at the end of the workday.	Having a healthy body is important to me and drinking isn't good for my body.	Switch the social drink for a trip to the gym or a walk.
2.		
3.		

MARSHMALLOWS IN RELATIONSHIPS

MARSHMALLOW IDENTIFIED	HOW THIS TAKES ME AWAY FROM MY TRUE NORTH	SMALL STEP I CAN TAKE TO SAY "NOT NOW"
1. Example: Constantly checking my cell phone when I'm out to dinner.	Family and friends matter to me and not being present when I'm with them is not respectful.	Leave my phone in the car or in my purse.
2.		
3.		

MARSHMALLOWS IN HEALTH/EXERCISE

MARSHMALLOW IDENTIFIED	HOW THIS TAKES ME AWAY FROM MY TRUE NORTH	SMALL STEP I CAN TAKE TO SAY "NOT NOW"
1. Example: Eating dessert every night after dinner.	I value good health and eating sugar every night is not healthy.	I am allowed to have dessert on Saturday nights only.
2.		
3.		

Step 4. PRACTICE DELAYING GRATIFICATION. Pick one area of your life: work, home, relationships, or health/exercise. Pick the biggest, tastiest marshmallow from that category, the one that would seem hardest to give up. Facebook? Beer? TV? Up to you. Next, pick a difficulty level you'd like to try:

_____ Delay gratification for 3 to 5 days.
_____ Delay gratification for 6 to 8 days.
_____ Delay gratification for 9 to 12 days.

Do it!

Gauge your self-control success. Track your marshmallows and identify what you've gained each week by delaying gratification.

DAY	MARSHMALLOW	WHAT I'VE GAINED
SUNDAY		
MONDAY		
TUESDAY		
WEDNESDAY		
THURSDAY		
FRIDAY		
SATURDAY		

MASTER CLASS

Barry Sternlicht, longtime real estate mogul, and founder, chairman, and CEO of Starwood Capital Group

AVOID INSTANT GRATIFICATION

At thirty, I got fired from my job. So I started a company with a couple of friends from school. We did a lot of things in the inverse. For example, we took no fees from investors until they got their money back. So they liked that, and we've kept that structure for twenty-three years. Our management fees just basically covered our salaries, which were modest, and we took it all at the end if we did well for the investors. You don't get anywhere without hard work and accountability.

"Perseverance is genius in disguise." I actually found that in a fortune cookie when I was in high school, which I kept in my wallet for eight years until I lost my wallet. I think the key is just picking yourself up off the ground, bucking adversity, because the world will knock you down. Life is not a straight line. I was collecting unemployment benefits when I was thirty-one, but I just kept looking forward, not back.

Find the freight trains in your life and get on them instead of in front of them. It sounds silly, but it really is important. Explore what's going to be a trend in your lifetime—technology, innovation, clean living, and healthy food? It's easier to go with the flow than against it, and if they match with your interests then that's an easy career.

Hope isn't a business strategy. You've got to make things happen. And you can. Everyone has twenty-four hours in the day and how you choose to use them is up to you. It's a fair world, right? I always wanted to make enough money so that I wouldn't have to worry about things for my kids, so that they could do whatever they want, and we could just be happy. I've accomplished that, but I keep going. Why? It's a little bit like a shark—if they stop swimming, they die! So I keep going. It's what I do. It's like my sport—in this I'm pretty good!

Luck is when preparation meets opportunity. So you create your own luck. Of course, you'll make mistakes along the way but you have to recognize them and keep going. I look at financing and investing like everything else in life—it has mechanical failure and pilot error. And I'm okay with mechanical failure. For example, we couldn't stop the financial crisis. But I'm not happy with the mistakes that we made. So you just retool yourself and you learn a lot. We learned a lot from the crisis, and there were some really grim days.

Even when it's grim, other's have seen worse. My dad was a Holocaust survivor. When your father is nine when the Nazis throw him out of his home, and his father, your grandfather, is sent to a Russian work camp, whatever you're going through doesn't compare. Whenever you think it's bad, you know it could always be much worse.

MAXIMIZE YOUR TIME

(SPARTAN VIRTUE: PRIORITIZATION)

If time be of all things most precious, wasting time must be the greatest prodigality, since lost time is never found again.

—BENJAMIN FRANKLIN

Seize the hour.

—SOPHOCLES

I hate to waste time. If I'm stuck somewhere, waiting for a flight or for my car to be repaired, I'll do burpees or push-ups to fill the gap. I don't care what people think. I find a way to make downtime count. You don't get much time in this life, so I want to squeeze every bit I can out of it while I'm here. William Penn wrote, "Time is what we want most, but what we spend worst." How true is that? I'm always conjuring up ways to spend time better. If you want to live the Spartan Way, you have to maximize the time you devote to getting to your True North. Otherwise, you'll spend a lot of time on stuff of little value. Prioritize what's important to you.

When I was in the construction business in the early nineties and someone came by looking for a job, I would literally hand them a shovel. "Come on," I'd say. "I'm going to interview you while we work." And you know what? That's a great way to get to know what someone is like, what they're made of: Hand him a shovel or a pick ax.

When you're on a construction job, you don't have the luxury of time to waste. You make the most of every second, and you make sure your labor knows this, too. Otherwise, you're losing money. No matter what business you're in, time is your most precious commodity. Every moment, every day, month, or year that we let slip by is a waste of what little time we have. That's why understanding how to manage time is one of the most useful principles you'll master on your Spartan journey.

Start by analyzing how much time you waste over the course of a day. If you say you don't have time to exercise, prepare healthier meals, or play with your kids, you're probably not being honest with yourself. You *can* find time. You're just not looking hard enough.

Try this: Spend the day with a small notebook and a pencil in your pocket. Every hour or two, jot down what you've accomplished in the last 60 to 120 minutes. Were you efficient? Where was the time wasted? How much of your day was spent chit-chatting, texting, surfing the web, eating chips, watching TV, or doing a zillion other mindless things that don't move you forward. What important tasks are you avoiding by occupying yourself with stuff that doesn't matter? Be brutally honest. Otherwise, you're wasting your time. At the end of the day, review your notes. It'll be an eye-opener. Most people who do this exercise, find at least an hour, sometimes two or more, *bonus hours* in their day. It's like finding free money.

Recently, I read an article in *Forbes* about time wasted on the job.

Of 750 employees who responded to a survey by Salary.com, 89 percent admitted to wasting time at work every day. Sixty-one percent said they wasted thirty minutes to an hour while 22 percent wasted two to three hours. Four percent admitted to wasting four to five hours! What the hell were they doing instead of their jobs? Salary.com asked that, too. The responses were:

- Talking on their phones or texting: 50 percent

- Gossiping: 42 percent

- On the internet: 39 percent

- On social media: 38 percent

- Taking snack or smoke breaks: 27 percent

It drives me nuts when I hear about time waste like that. I'm thinking: "These lazy asses at least could have been doing burpees!"

See my point? We waste time on the job and commuting an hour each way. We waste it at home. And yet we complain that we have no time. Well, go ahead and do that little time-analysis exercise. You will find more than enough time to accomplish everything you say you don't have time to get done.

The trick to effective time management is discipline. It goes back to what you learned in Principle #1, Find Your True North and Principle #2, Make a Commitment. When you know your purpose, you're driven to make the best use of your time to pursue it. When you make a dedicated commitment, you've already decided to say "no" to stuff that competes for your time. Binge-watch *Game of Thrones* or go for your scheduled ten-mile run? No contest. Go out to the bar with friends or study for a final in an MBA course? You'll either make the time to do both or you'll blow off your buddies until next time. See, time management isn't that difficult when you have your priorities straight.

SWEAT EQUITY

Here's a story about how committing to my True North priorities helps me maximize every moment. You know what my priorities are, right? Health, Family, Work, Fun, in that order. Okay, so two guys I had met several years ago during a Death Race call me up and ask for a meeting to discuss a business idea. They want to talk in person, but the problem is I'm in Ithaca taking my boys to a wrestling camp. It's seven and a half hours away for these guys. That's okay, they say, they'll drive.

Now, these guys know me, so they show up at 6 a.m. fully expecting there will be two one-hundred-pound rocks with their names on them and a note telling them to carry it five miles to the next clue about my location. (That's not out of character, actually; I've done things like that.)

This time, however, I'm there in flesh and blood. But it's time for my ten-mile run and I've made a commitment to put my health first without deviation. So I say: "Let's run and talk."

We take off but don't get much talking done. When we finish the run, it's time for my pull-ups: 150. They do them, too. Our hands are bleeding. Might as well get the burpees done, I tell them. We set a timer for seventy-second bouts of burpees. I don't tell them we're doing three hundred. Actually, we lose count and do more.

And still, we haven't had a chance to talk business. I suggest we walk to breakfast. The diner is twenty minutes down the road. After the meal, I'm on phone meetings for two and a half hours. And these guys are waiting patiently. It's one o'clock before we have a chance to talk in earnest—seven hours after they drove seven and a half hours. My point is, I didn't let their agenda change my agenda. My workout and work time are non-negotiable. Nothing gets in the way of the path to my True North.

And those two Death Race guys? Man, they met me every step of the way without complaint. They showed me they understand commitment. I didn't even have to listen to their pitch. Whatever their idea is, if they show that kind of drive, I know they're gonna crush it.

ANOTHER BIG TIME SUCK

There's another place where we waste a huge amount of time besides the TV set and the internet. Karl Pillemer, PhD, a professor of gerontology at Cornell University's College of Human Ecology, discovered it in the course of his research with the Legacy Project. This guy goes around collecting practical advice for better living from people who've earned the knowledge—America's elderly folks. In one segment of the project, Pillemer asked more than twelve hundred people over the age of sixty-five what they regretted most when they looked back on their lives. The most common answer? "Worrying too much." They realized too late that they wasted so much of life fretting over events they couldn't control. Their advice on overcoming this was pretty direct: Train yourself, no matter how, to eliminate, or at least reduce, worry, and do more important things with the time that you have.

Dr. Pillemer hit on a big one there. Worry is a huge time suck. It's the repetition of a thought pattern that never resolves a situation. We only think it might. Chronic worriers believe they can prevent a bad thing from happening if they worry about it enough. Of course, worrying is not proactive at all, and Pillemer's elderly subjects learned this the hard way. Plus, chronic worry goes hand in hand with anxiety disorders and depression and it can lead to substance abuse. The lesson here is that worry is worthless. Use your True North to set and stick to your priorities. Do what matters first.

PRIORITY 1

Like me, you're probably too young to remember our thirty-fourth president, Dwight David Eisenhower, who was known as Ike. In a famous speech given in 1954 to the Second Assembly of the World Council of Churches, Ike said, "I have two kinds of problems, the urgent and the important. The urgent are not important and the important are never urgent."

Eisenhower was a master of planning and a prolific doer. As the Allied Forces' Supreme Commander during World War II and later president, Eisenhower made dozens of tough decisions daily. He didn't have time for worry. He needed solutions. Eisenhower came to believe that, in many cases, we prioritize tasks that we believe are urgent and ignore those that truly are critical to success. This led him to develop a principle that helps prioritize tasks by urgency and importance. In what became known as The Eisenhower Matrix or The Eisenhower Box, Ike illustrated a solution to a problem that we all face: Deciding where to focus our efforts amid a plethora of seemingly equal demands. The common problem it solves is indecisiveness and the time it wastes. When we spend too much of our time avoiding making a wrong decision, the fear makes us impotent to act and we run out of opportunities that could move us forward. Using Eisenhower's matrix makes organizing tasks easier by placing them into one of four possible boxes:

1. Urgent and important (tasks you will do immediately).

2. Important, but not urgent (tasks you will schedule to do later).

3. Urgent, but not important (tasks you will delegate to someone else).

4. Neither urgent nor important (tasks that you will eliminate).

Here's what the Eisenhower box looks like:

DO FIRST	SCHEDULE
First focus on important tasks to be done the same day.	Important, but not-so-urgent stuff should be scheduled.
DELEGATE	DON'T DO
What's urgent, but less important, delegate to others.	What's neither urgent nor important don't do at all.

There's more on the President Eisenhower's Box Method in "Get Off the Couch!" on page 105.

PULLED IN TOO MANY DIRECTIONS

I wish I had known about The Eisenhower Matrix sooner. Before I started Spartan, I was juggling way too many tasks, thinking that every one of them was equally important. I was competing in different ultra-events around the world. I was also putting together races for incredibly driven athletes.

I had left a solid job on Wall Street and moved my family to Vermont. Here, Courtney and I were busy building numerous businesses including a farm, a bed and breakfast, and a general store for hikers. We wanted to secure a stable future for our kids and were putting as many eggs in our basket as possible. The problem was, I was being pulled in all directions, trying to prioritize every task while advancing none of them. I knew my True North, but I was making life too complicated. I needed to take a step back, catch my breath, and think.

Important tasks are those that support our values, our beliefs, our True North. We approach them with more thought and thoroughness and less hurry than we do urgent tasks. We respond to them with logic rather than reacting to them with emotion.

I started to learn that urgent tasks are often associated with achieving someone else's goals. They're the ones the CEO is shouting at you to do. They're the ones that flash at you from the subject lines of your email in-box, written in caps or with a red *priority* signal attached. They are reactions you have to your Twitter feed, Facebook comments, and text messages. They scream for your attention because they'll deliver immediate results. They feel important. Typically, though, urgent tasks are nothing more than distractions dragging us further away from what's vital to our lives.

> With every decision, big or small, ask yourself, "Does this choice take me closer to my True North or further away from it?"

When I finally pulled back from juggling all my interests and putting everyone's needs before my own and I started Spartan Race, it meant dropping everything else. I put all my skin into a game that meant so much to me. And that's when things started to come together.

MASTER CLASS

Tim Ferriss, author of THE 4-HOUR WORKWEEK
and THE 4-HOUR BODY

I try to make the first part of my day, the three or four hours before lunch, uninterrupted—the "maker" or creative portion of my day. In the afternoon I'll do my phone calls and meetings, the management part of the day.

I have a journaling practice that I do for a few minutes in the morning and a few at night before bed. At night, I'll spec out the two or three objectives for the next day and two or three attributes that I want to exemplify for that day. One attribute I write down a lot is "unrushed." I also do a postgame analysis each night. It's one of my rituals.

My Morning Routine:

Wake up between 6:30 and 7:00 a.m.

Meditate for fifteen to twenty minutes repeating a word or sound.

Turn on Pandora and listen to some chill Brazilian music while journaling for five minutes.

Exercise: a series of mobility moves.

Writing, podcast work, and other creative tasks until lunchtime.

If I have a task I want to avoid, I'll give myself a little Scooby snack first thing. I'll do one or two fun items before I get into that most gnarly task. For instance, I'm trying to learn a new type of drum. So I take two minutes to set up my drum lesson. Okay, Scooby snack. Then I'm ready to get into the salt mines.

WILL IT MAKE THE BOAT GO FASTER?

Spartan Race's mission is to rip people off the couch and make them fit. To accomplish that mission, I knew I had to be truly Spartan, selfishly frugal with my time and energy. You must be frugal, too. With every decision, big or small, ask yourself, "Does this choice take me closer to my True North or further away from it?" This simple strategy will comb through your decisions, clearing out those unimportant ones that don't align with your goals. This strategy has roots in an Olympic story about the British men's rowing team that went from finishing near last at the Atlanta Olympics in 1996 to winning Olympic Gold four years later in Sydney. England's coxed eight team had consistently failed to medal or even make the finals in the major regattas. So they decided to change everything about their approach to training and working together. As the athletes prepared for the Sydney Games, the crew decided that they would ask themselves one clear and crucial question before undertaking any action either as a team or as individuals: *Will it make the boat go faster?*

Will extra training make the boat go faster? Yes.

Will putting more time on the rowing machine each day make the boat go faster? Yes.

Will partying on the weekend make the boat go faster? No.

For eighteen months, as they trained, these ordinary athletes answered yes or no to the question—*will it make the boat go faster?*—and on the day of the Olympic final, against all the odds, their boat went faster than any other boat in the race, and they took home their first Olympic title.

Everyone was shocked that the team had won, but those people were only looking at the rowers' previous race results. They didn't consider that the British crew had taken the time to identify what was truly important and had spent the last year and a half building on that. Their win didn't come down to some mad, urgent dash to the finish line. It began in the many months running up to the games as these athletes recognized how to effectively manage their time. Every seemingly insignificant decision along the way, when stacked on top of one another, led them to a gold medal. At the same time, because they relentlessly questioned their actions in relation to their goal, the British rowers weren't just prioritizing new actions; they were creating new habits.

BUILDING HABITS

Habits are central to prioritization. Bad habits take you away from your goal. Good habits bring you closer. But how do we develop good habits when bad habits keep distracting us? Fortunately, there is an easy strategy that has been proven effective in more than 100 studies on everything from time management to substance abuse to diet and exercise. Psychologists call it "implementation intention" but it's better known as "if-then planning." It's pretty simple: You decide in advance when and where you will do something specific that will advance you toward your goal. For example: Say your goal is to lose weight by cutting out doughnuts. Every time you start to reach for a doughnut or even think about a doughnut, you use that as a cue to drink a glass of cold water. The doughnut triggers a specific action—drinking water. *If I think about eating a doughnut, then I will drink a glass of cold water, instead.*

Psychologists say we humans are pretty good about remembering information and carrying out tasks when they are put in "If X, then Y" terms. In one study, researchers recruited people who wanted to start a regular exercise routine. Half of the participants were asked to create an If-Then Plan about when and where they would exercise three times each week. For example: "*If* it is Monday, Wednesday, or Friday, *then* I will go to the gym for an hour before work." The other half of the group did not use an If-Then Plan. The result? After several months, 91 percent of the if-then planners were still exercising, compared to just 39 percent of the non-planners.

This is how you build your habit using If-Then Planning: Create a cue or trigger (the "if") that reminds you to initiate an action (the "then") that ultimately rewards you. The more positive the reward, the more closely tied it is to an important goal or dream, the more you'll want to repeat this cycle. For the British rowing team, their persistent question "Will it make the boat go faster?" became the cue that helped them create a routine that would finally deliver the reward that they all craved—winning an Olympic medal for their country.

The more successful your habits are, the more effortless the task you're carrying out becomes. You just do it. You get out of bed when the alarm goes off, you go to the gym, you do your daily burpees, you spend time with your loved ones, you make those calls and push those sales that keep you in business. You do what's important because it's habit. Many people say they can never find the time to work out. What they mean is that they haven't made working out a priority. They haven't made it a habit so that they can deliver on their promise to themselves.

You will obviously have different cues depending on the habit you're trying to form. If your goal is to be a better partner and parent, your cue might be the sound of your kids arriving home from school or your partner's car pulling up in the driveway. You close down your laptop, put aside what you were doing, and you concentrate on being fully present for them.

If you're building your own business, creating strong habits can steady your path to success. In a conversation with entrepreneur and author Tim Ferriss, he told me that he has a number of daily habits that enable him to prioritize what is important for him to achieve that day. For starters, he narrows his daily "to-do" list down to one or two items. He also blocks out his morning to do active tasks such as writing, planning, and creating. Then in the afternoon, he concentrates more on management-related, reactive tasks such as telephone calls, sending emails, and meetings.

Tim also has a habit of doing two or three quick, fun tasks first thing before he rolls up his sleeves to tackle the more challenging assignments. He calls these Scooby Snacks and they act as cues to help him launch into his day with greater enthusiasm.

This idea of connecting something fun or a reward with something challenging has also been investigated in relation to forming exercise habits. The problem with so many people is that, on an intellectual level, they know that maintaining a regular workout is going to make them healthier, happier, and add years to their lives. But on a motivational level—they're just not feeling it. Alison Phillips, an assistant professor of psychology at Iowa State University, found the solution. She put together a study that analyzed activity levels for individuals beginning to work out, and those who had been exercising regularly for at least three months. The results showed that those who needed that extra prod were more successful at keeping an exercise habit when they combined a cue with an intrinsic reward.

So what does that involve? First, you need to create a cue that triggers the exercise behavior, such as an alarm going off when it's time to hit the gym, say, or a reminder note stuck to your bathroom mirror to drop and do three burpees every time you finish washing your hands.

Secondly, you have to work on encoding intrinsic rewards associated with the specific benefits that you'll reap from engaging in exercise. This is a little more difficult. It takes time and trial and error. No two people will be equally inspired by the same inner reward. Your reward has to have a

MASTER CLASS

Ben Greenfield, exercise physiologist, coach, and author of BEYOND TRAINING

DO WHAT'S IMPORTANT FIRST

One reason I do hard things is because I want to raise amazing human beings who are going to grow up and make this world a better place. I want to be able to inspire my kids and, in order to do that, I have to be the strongest version of me. I can't allow other activities to take me away from what's important.

I train with my family. My wife and I put our kids on our backs and do hill sprints. We love exercising with our kids. Studies have shown that when kids see parents who are fit and physically active, they automatically become more active.

I have this favorite hike I love to do with my kids. I'll wear a weighted vest and one of those elevation-training masks that restrict airflow so it's like you're breathing through a straw. People look at me like "that's a little strange," but I think strange is good. It's okay to be unique. Makes life interesting. Besides, I have a great workout, I get to hang out with my kids, and they get to hang out with me. If you want to get something done, make it a priority, and make it fun.

personal meaning to you. To figure out what is intrinsically most rewarding about an exercise, try to connect with yourself every time you complete a physical activity to see what benefits you gained. You might say, "I felt so fed-up and exhausted before I went for a run but now I feel really energized and fired-up." This feeling of energy is the intrinsic reward that keeps you coming back for more. Equally, you might say, "I was stressed before I went hill-walking with my dog, now I feel completely calm and rested." Again, dog plus hill-walking equals motivation to move your ass. Other experiments have proven that anticipating a reward releases a rush of dopamine, the neurochemical that mediates pleasure in the brain. So by linking exercise with something that's already rewarding for you—like a walk with your dog—your brain begins to look forward to it.

GET OFF THE COUCH!
How to Maximize Your Time

Step 1. ELIMINATE PERFECTIONISM TO DEFEAT PROCRASTINATION.
Feeling inadequate breeds procrastination. Take the example of the tennis player who feels he's not quite good enough yet to join a singles league. He needs a new pair of tennis shoes and the *right* racquet. He thinks he needs another lesson, needs to read another book, or watch another technique video. He gets so caught up in having everything perfect and ignores the most critical step: Doing the work and playing the game.
Ask yourself:

"Where am I spending 90 percent of my time versus doing the work?"
"Where am I procrastinating?"
"How am I putting off doing the work?"
"What fears are keeping me from taking first steps toward my goal?"

After you gain clarity, start making better use of your time by— you guessed it—doing the work.

Step 2. MANAGE YOUR TIME BEFORE IT MANAGES YOU. You only have about twelve waking hours each day to make things happen. The rest of the twenty-four-hour clock is spent either sleeping, eating, dressing, commuting, etc. And as you move through the day, your window for doing things gets smaller and smaller. To make each moment count, you need to be selfish about your time. Review that notebook I recommended that you keep. Ask yourself: "Is what I'm doing right now leading to my True North?" "Will this help me achieve my goal?" "Will it make *my boat* go faster?" If the answer is *yes,* go for it. If it's *no,* switch to something that will.

Step 3. ORGANIZE YOUR PRIORITIES WITH THE EISENHOWER BOX. Start by making a list of all the tasks you want to complete in a day or week. Be realistic. Keep the list to about eight items or less. If you load it up with fifteen to twenty tasks, the list will feel overwhelming, not to mention impossible to complete. Next, rate the tasks by placing them into one of the four boxes.

Box 1. Tasks are those that would cause significant problems for you if you didn't complete them.

Box 2. Tasks listed here are important but not urgent. Schedule them for later, after urgent tasks have been completed.

Box 3. In this box, list tasks that don't need your skills. Delegate these tasks. They are a waste of your time and can be handled by others.

Box 4. In this quadrant, place tasks like mindless Facebook browsing, watching TV reruns, and things that aren't at all necessary to your profession, health, and relational life.

	Urgent	Not Urgent
Important	**I** Activities: Crises Pressing problems Deadline-driven projects	**II** Activities: Prevention Relationship building Recreation New opportunities
Not Important	**III** Activities: Interruptions Some phone calls Some mail Some meetings Popular activities	**IV** Activities: Trivia Some mail Some phone calls Time wasters Pleasure activities

Step 4. CREATE AN IF-THEN PLAN TO BUILD HABITS. Determine a cue (the "If") that triggers you to perform a specific behavior (the "then"). Examples: If I see my running shoes near the door, then I will go for a run. If I want a snack, I'll grab a piece of fruit. If I'm waiting around for something, I'll use the time productively by doing 10 burpees or 30 air squats. Choose your cue wisely. It needs to be powerful enough to trigger the desired behavior.

Burpees >

THE MOST TIME-EFFICIENT EXERCISE IN THE WORLD
(And Arguably the Most Badass)

If you can't find the time in your day for a workout, give me thirty burpees. It exercises your entire body, your heart, and your lungs. It's efficient and it taxes your body like no other exercise. That's why if you fail to make it through a Spartan Race obstacle, your penalty is thirty burpees before you can move on. You don't get a pass. Burpees are an excuse-buster.

The burpee is a version of the squat thrust you did in eighth-grade gym class. It's my favorite exercise because:

1. You can do it just about anywhere and you need only your body—no equipment—and only a 2-by-6-foot patch of ground.
2. It's total body exercise that builds athleticism, which incorporates flexibility, quickness, agility, coordination, endurance, strength, and power. Plus, burpees burn a shitload of calories.

In one fitness study, ROTC cadets were given a test that measures anaerobic power and capacity. Half of the cadets performed four rounds of thirty-second all-out sprints on a stationary cycle with four-minute rests in between. The other group did thirty-second rounds of burpees. Both high-intensity workouts were equally effective at cranking metabolism, but the cadets who did burpees felt the effects all over their bodies, not just their legs and lungs. Another study published in the *Journal of Strength and Conditioning Research* analyzed and ranked the metabolic responses of thirteen different types of free-weight resistance, bodyweight, and battling rope exercises. Burpees came in second place only to battling rope exercises in lung-searing metabolic demand.

Do a Spartan Standard Race Burpee and think about how many incredible fitness elements you get in one total-body movement:

From a standing position, squat and place your hands on the ground in front of you. The squat is arguably the single best exercise known to man. Do squats all your life and you will never need assistance getting out of chair to blow out the 101 candles on your birthday cake.

Kick your legs straight out behind you and assume the top of a push-up position. You're in a plank, one of the best moves for building core strength.

Do a push-up. Bend your arms to lower your torso until your chest touches the ground and then straighten your arms to push yourself back up. This builds upper body strength.

Jump both feet forward between your hands, keeping your hips high. This is a dynamic stretch for your hips, hamstrings, quads, lower back, and shoulders.

Press your feet into the ground to jump explosively straight up in the air and clap your hands together overhead. This plyometric movement builds leg strength and explosive power. Plus, the rapid-fire nature of burpee reps drives cardiovascular conditioning and boosts metabolism on par with the toughest *high-intensity interval training* (HIIT) workouts.

To the woman and man who claim to have no time for exercise, the burpee responds: "No excuse. Period."

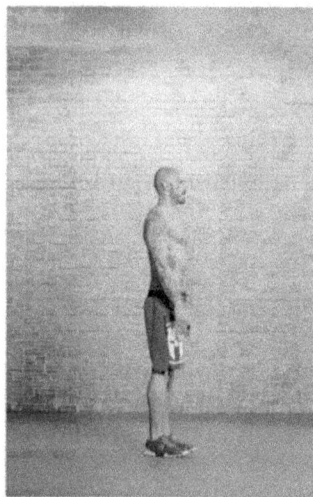

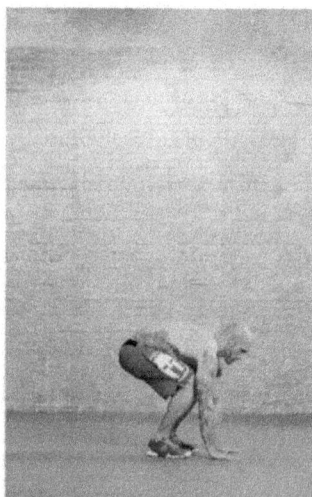

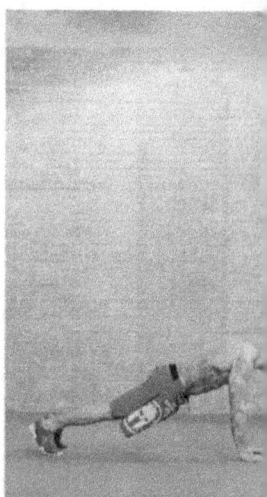

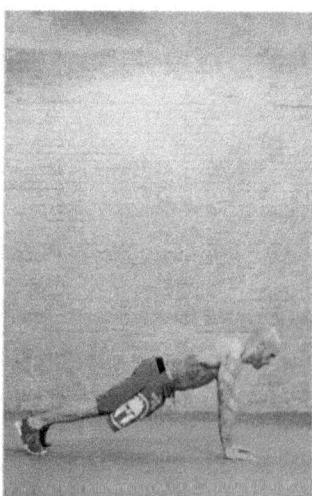

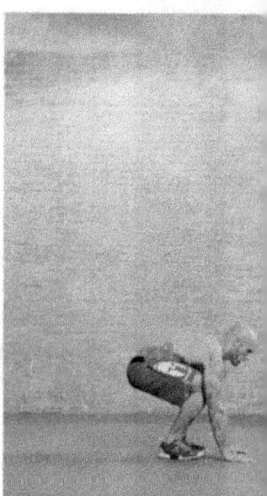

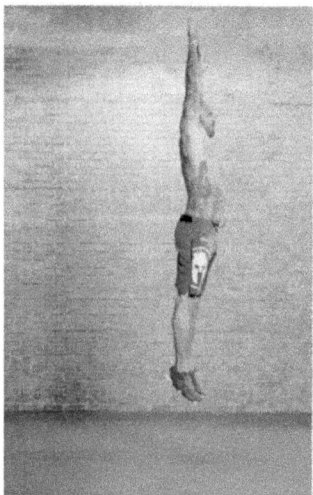

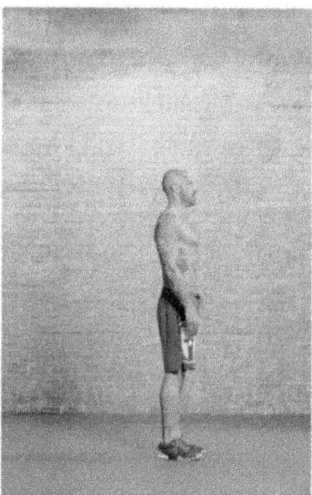

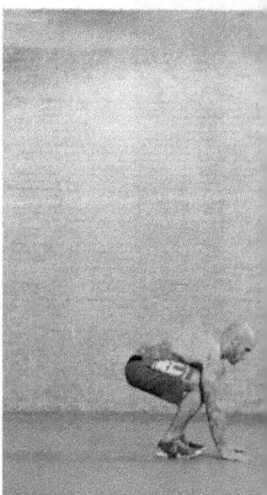

PRINCIPLE #6

GET GRITTY

(SPARTAN VIRTUE: GRIT)

> The credit belongs to the man who is actually in the arena, whose face is marred
> by dust and sweat and blood; who strived valiantly; who errs, who comes short again and
> again . . . who at the best knows in the end the triumph of high achievement, and who at
> the worst, if he fails, at least fails while daring greatly.
>
> —TEDDY ROOSEVELT

> It is better to be a lion for a day than a sheep all your life.
>
> —SISTER ELIZABETH KENNY

Grit is the ability to stay motivated even when the shit is flying and you're covered in it. When you face failure after failure and you crawl in a hole to lick your wounds; grit is the tenacity that makes you crawl back out.

Grit is elusive. It's one of the hardest Spartan traits to build but one of the most powerful. You might have encountered grit in twelfth-grade English class while reading Tennyson's "Ulysses." In the famous last line of that poem, Tennyson describes Ulysses and his mariners as "strong in will," sustained by their resolve to push on relentlessly, "To strive, to seek, to find, *and not to yield.*"

That's grit.

Grit is something you have to work on all your life. I started my education in grit early on and I'm still learning.

I LOVE TEXTILES!

I wasn't what you'd call a high achiever in high school, so I had no business applying to Cornell University. But a friend of mine said, "Hey, my dad's a professor; he'll get us in." I figured that's the way it worked in my old neighborhood—you had a connection, it got you places. I didn't know any better, so I said, "Okay, let's go to Cornell."

We both did interviews and thought we totally crushed them. Obviously, I'm not the smartest guy in the room. We were both denied. My buddy's dad sat us down and told us that if we took some classes elsewhere and did well, we could build up credits and reapply.

I suggested to my friend that we go back to Queens, work on my pool business, and take classes at St. John's to learn how to study. "Great plan," he said, "but I'm going to Vegas. If I have to buckle down in the fall, I want to party all summer." (His response helped me learn another valuable principle, about delaying gratification. At St. John's, I studied the marshmallow test. If I can wait—not go to Vegas to have fun—I can have a better life.)

I studied hard at St. John's and reapplied to Cornell. I was rejected. I applied again. I was rejected again. I felt pretty beat up and contemplated packing it in and focusing on my pool business. But I decided to apply a fourth time. Perseverance has a way of paying off, often through strange opportunities. At the time I was planning to reapply, my mother told me she was teaching yoga to a Cornell professor, who was willing to meet with me. Professor Anita Racine was the Director of Undergraduate Studies in the Department of Textiles & Apparel. "I have ninety-two women enrolled, but no men," she told me. Then she asked, "Do you like textiles?"

"Yeah, I love textiles and I am designing and selling T-shirts!"

That's how I got into Cornell.

All of us can use more grit. I've been fascinated by the idea of cultivating grit for years. So, when I read this amazing book called *Grit: The Power of Passion and Perseverance,* I had to visit the author. Angela Duckworth, PhD, is a psychology professor and MacArthur "genius" fellow at the University of Pennsylvania. She also runs a nonprofit called Character Lab.

Duckworth told me she started looking into this character trait when she was a seventh-grade math teacher in the New York's public school system. She noticed something interesting: Many of her smartest students performed terribly on the SATs, while less talented kids scored the best. She became fascinated with exploring what made some people, in stressful situations, more successful than others.

Duckworth went to graduate school to study psychology and research this puzzling phenomenon. She visited schools in rough neighborhoods to see which new teachers would be first to quit and which would suck it up and stay. She attended the National Spelling Bee and studied the kids who were more likely to advance through the competition. Then, she went to West Point, where she watched America's most promising students get their asses kicked building resilience and leadership skills during Cadet Basic Training, better known as "Beast Barracks" or just "Beast." She was curious about the character traits of students who survive the seven-week ordeal.

Most psychologists assumed that the men and women who made it through Beast were the very smart ones who came to the academy with the highest GPAs, class ranks, and SAT scores. But Duckworth suspected something different. She found that the best predictor of success was not a cadet's intelligence but his or her ability to complete long-term demanding goals. In other words: Grit.

Duckworth defines grit as "passion and perseverance for very long-term goals." "People who are gritty," she told me, "are incredibly, doggedly tenacious about a singular goal. They don't just put in consistent effort but maintain focused interest over time."

The cadets who Duckworth predicted would make it through Beast scored highest on what she calls "the grit scale," a tick-the-box test with statements like "I don't give up easily" and "I have overcome setbacks to conquer an important challenge." People who think that way see life as a marathon, not a sprint, Duckworth says. They're committed for the long haul. *Committed,* not merely *interested.* Gritty people don't lose it in the face of adversity and plateaus. Disappointment or boredom won't signal them to cut their losses and change direction. They stay the course.

This may seem obvious: Work hard, stay focused, and be successful. Not exactly breaking news. But the fact is that most people don't believe that hard work beats natural genius or talent. A management researcher at University College London studied this phenomenon in an experiment. She presented the people in her study with two hypothetical entrepreneurs, one striving to succeed and the other who emphasized his natural ability. Then she asked participants to judge how successful they thought each would become based on a description of both entrepreneurs and listening to a one-minute clip of their business ideas. It turned out that most participants believed that the hypothetical entrepreneur with innate talent would be more successful.

Angela Duckworth sees our belief that born-in talent trumps years of committed effort as a cop-out, our way of shrugging off the responsibility to become the best that we can be. "We want to believe that Mark Spitz was born to swim in a way that none of us were and that none of us could," she says. "We don't want to sit on the pool deck and watch him progress from amateur to expert. We prefer our excellence fully formed. We prefer mystery to mundanity."

It's a mark of our own insecurity, Duckworth explains. If we don't believe we've been bestowed with the talent to compete, then we don't have to compete, and then we can't fail. In this way, our brains rationalize taking the easy way out. I agree, but I think laziness works its way in there, too. As the American writer, George Edward Woodberry, said, "Defeat is not the worst of failures. Not to have tried is the true failure."

When I think of gritty people, I picture Thomas Edison. He made one thousand attempts to create a lightbulb before he actually succeeded. I'm sure some friend along the way said, "Jeez, Tom, you've tried seventy-five times already, don't you think you should give it up?" Edison didn't listen. Or I think of the first woman to swim across the English Channel. Gertrude Ederle was just nineteen years old. This was in 1926. It was her second attempt. She faced twenty-foot waves and killer jellyfish and swam the channel two hours faster than any man had up until then. Her record stood until 1951. Somebody asked her how she did it. She said, "I knew it could be done; it had to be done, and I did it."

That's it. That's grit.

So how do *you* build the Spartan virtue of grit? How do you remain committed to your True North when you're being pounded by adversity and receiving body blow after body blow of bad luck?

Duckworth has a recipe. She says the four ingredients for grit are *passion, practice, purpose,* and *hope.* As you've already learned in this book, identifying your passion and following your True North are vital to success. Sometimes you have a lot of passions, as I did: The pool

> # MASTER CLASS
> **Mark Divine, former Navy SEAL, author of**
> THE WAY OF THE SEAL and UNBEATABLE MIND, and
> **founder of SEALFIT**
>
>
> Most people don't realize that their life is made up of the quality of the small choices they make moment to moment; it's rarely by the big choices that confront them. The essence of mental toughness is to develop enough control so that you can notice those choices *when* you are making them, especially wrong choices. When you can pause long enough in your mental space where time is irrelevant, then you can eliminate that wrong option and choose a new path.
>
> The most important lesson for mental toughness, then, is to know your *why*. Why are you here? If you are super-clear about why you are doing the thing, then in every moment when the going gets tough and you get kicked in the balls, you can say, "This is okay because I know why I'm doing it and it's worth it."

business, Wall Street, and endurance racing. That's okay. Looking back, I see a *through line* that links all these interests in my life, a line that also empowered me to develop grit along the way.

Barry Hearn, the founder of Matchroom Sport, calls this a scattergun approach. "Try it all. Eventually, you'll recognize the limitations within yourself that'll point you to your real passion," he said to me when we got talking about this stuff at a meeting in London. "Then go after it like a pit bull on a steak."

Hearn wanted to be the heavyweight-boxing champion of the world when he was a kid. His hero was Muhammad Ali. He grew up poor in the tenements of London's East End and had to raise his siblings after his dad died young. But this didn't stop him from chasing his dream. He trained hard and studied the boxing greats. He was relentless. "But I finally realized I wasn't good enough, so I became something else—a boxing promoter."

Hearn didn't give up his love of the sport. Instead, he found another way to follow his *passion*. Did it work out for him? Well, he's now a multimillionaire who claims every working day of his life has been a pleasure. What do you think?

Once you find your passion, cultivate it by continuously exploring its different levels and dimensions through *practice*, Duckworth's second ingredient. Keep your interest fired up by challenging yourself and pushing harder. Want to run a marathon? Not going to happen unless you get out and run long distances. Want to become a concert pianist? Sit down at the piano and start playing until your fingers bleed. Want to be a better parent? Cut the crap and practice being one.

When Duckworth studied kids who aced their regional Spelling Bee contest to make it to national finals, she discovered that the grittiest competitors turned in hours of practice. But they didn't just practice difficult words. They identified the words that tripped them up all the time and focused on practicing those. This was the same for the grittier West Point cadets. They persisted in practicing and overcoming the activities at which they didn't excel, not the ones they could crush.

Experts call this "deliberate practice." It involves rolling up your sleeves and expending considerable sweat practicing the skill you suck at until what once felt like failure is executed with fluency and finesse. Hungarian psychologist Mihaly Csikszentmihalyi (pronounced cheekssent-me-high) calls this level of mastery and intention *flow*. It's the feeling of being *in the zone,* so absorbed with what you're doing that nothing else matters and time seems to stand still. But a moment of flow can't happen without hours of practice. As Duckworth says, people like to believe that exceptional individuals were born with the innate abilities of a superhero. However, studies show that the characteristics once believed to reflect natural talent are the result of intense practice, at least twenty hours a week over a minimum of ten years. In his book *Outliers,* Malcolm Gladwell describes something similar, the "10,000-hour rule." He argues that it takes about ten thousand hours of practice for someone to achieve real mastery of any skill. So you may want to dust off that ukelele in the corner and start practicing again.

Part of learning through deliberate practice is learning through constant feedback. It doesn't matter if it's negative. Use it to figure out and fix what's going wrong. Then apply your learning to practicing again and again and again. The Japanese have a word for this in business. They call it "Kaizen," the philosophy of continuous improvement.

Following practice, the third characteristic that gritty people share is a sense of *purpose.* When the ancient Spartans entered battle they weren't just fighting for their own lives, but the lives of all their brother soldiers. They found this purpose through years of training and living side by side in the *agoge.*

Developing a sense of purpose beyond the self is possible for all of us because we're social creatures. Back in prehistoric times, those who united in small groups were more likely to survive than those who chose to go it alone. In modern society that connection and need to support and protect community is just as strong. We all have that urge inside of us.

My mission for Spartan is to jump-start millions of individuals into living active, fit lives. And I know that one of the best ways to do that is by helping people experience the camaraderie of an adventure race where fellow Spartans to your left and right help you to climb over obstacles if you're struggling. A Spartan race is an amazing experience because it's a shared experience that generates mutual respect.

Hope, or optimism, is the final variable in Duckworth's grit formula. It's probably the most crucial because it's about interpreting and dealing with setbacks. Richard Branson, the Virgin Atlantic mogul, is a guy who credits his optimistic attitude with helping him overcome tons of setbacks. When I met with him, we talked about his balloon-flying failures. He spent a large part of his life attempting to be the first across the Atlantic, and then the Pacific, in a hot-air balloon. I didn't know he had landed in the sea around five times and had to be rescued by helicopter. I was really struck by the positive way he viewed each failed voyage. "Nobody had attempted it before," he said. "And if you're going to do something that hasn't been done before, you have to accept that it's going to be difficult."

> **God helps those who persevere.**
>
> —Koran
>
> **He that endureth to the end shall be saved.**
>
> —Matthew 10:22

Branson earned the record for both the first Atlantic and Pacific crossings and came within one day of being the first to go around the world in a hot-air balloon.

"We hit this blanket of air off America and we couldn't get through," he said. "But the truth is that it didn't matter. The satisfaction we got was in trying these things, these incredible adventures. We learned that it was the attempt that mattered more."

Developing a hopeful or optimistic outlook on life is a learned behavior. Purpose and practice can prod you toward cultivating hopefulness. I like to say, "Smile through it and see what happens." Being positive is a lot more fun than the alternative.

WHAT I'VE LEARNED

Ricardo "The Animal" Migliarese, first-degree Jiu-Jitsu black belt, national and world champion

Ricardo Migliarese grew up the target of ruthless bullies on the mean streets of South Philly and transformed raw toughness into something that could help others. He and his brother Phil teach Gracie Brazilian Jiu-Jitsu, mixed martial arts, and yoga for fighters at Balance Studios in Philadelphia.

As a kid I was on the street hanging with the worst of the worst and I got to see who the tough guys really were. It wasn't those guys.

My father taught us to play chess. Jiu-Jitsu is pretty much physical chess.

Jiu-Jitsu is something you're never the best at. You can do it all your life and keep learning. I have a seventy-year-old who is blind who trains with us.

I love the pull-up. There's a lot of pull action in Jiu-Jitsu. I do a one-hundred-rep workout all different ways. When my daughter turned one, I did 325 pull-ups.

Jiu-Jitsu is a lifestyle. It's about trying to change people's lives. I teach my heart out. My goal is to have my students tap me out.

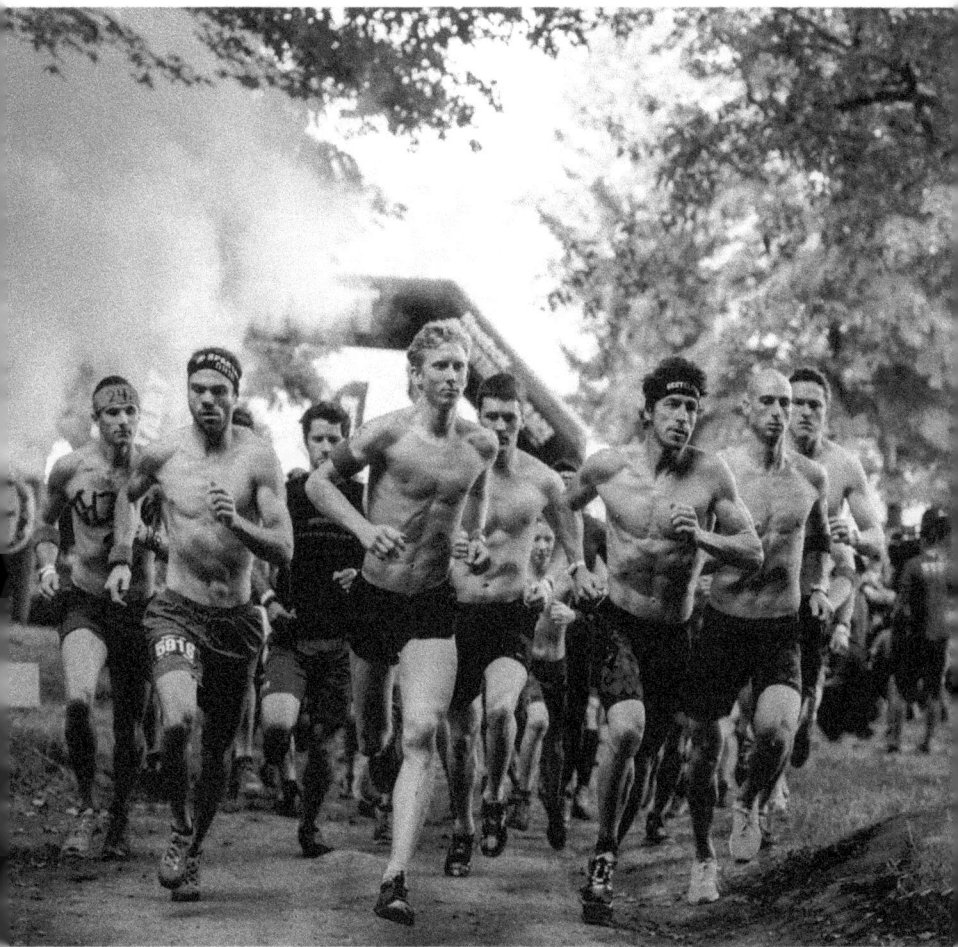

Elite male athletes at the start of the 2014 "Spartan Pac West Sprint" in Washougal, WA.

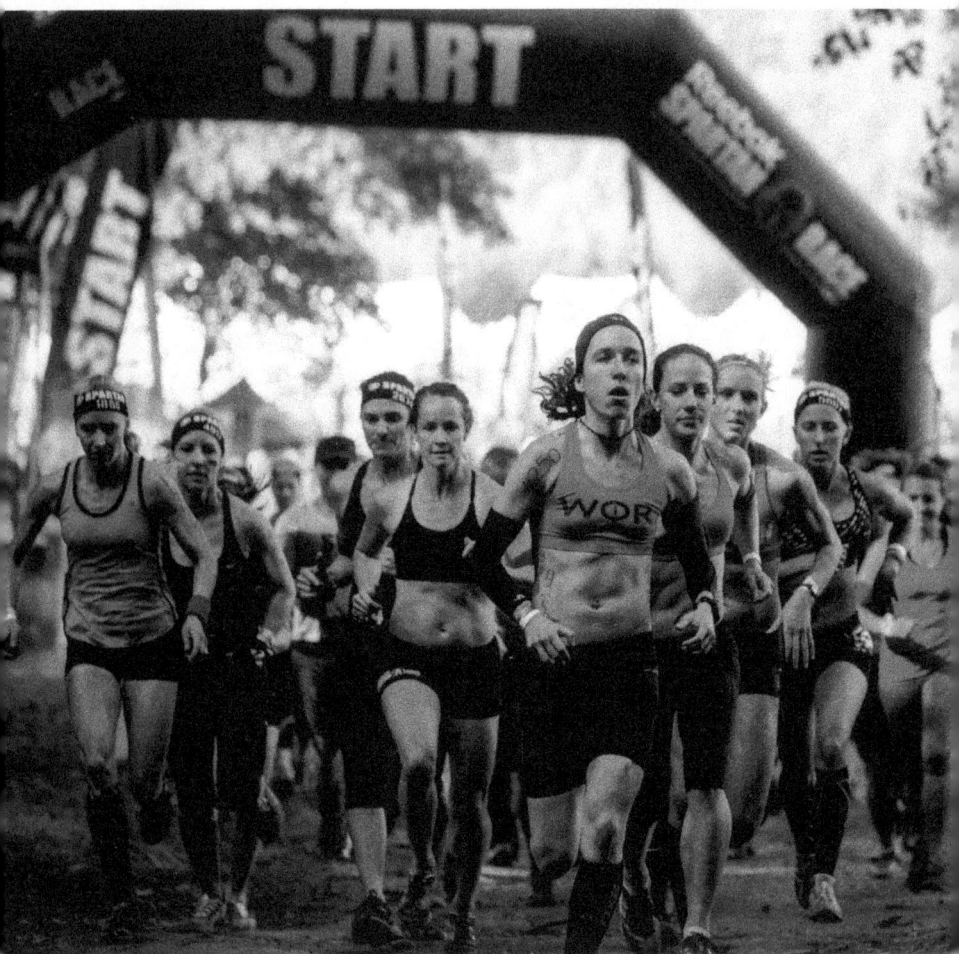

Elite female athletes at the start of the 2014 "Spartan Pac West Sprint" in Washougal, WA.

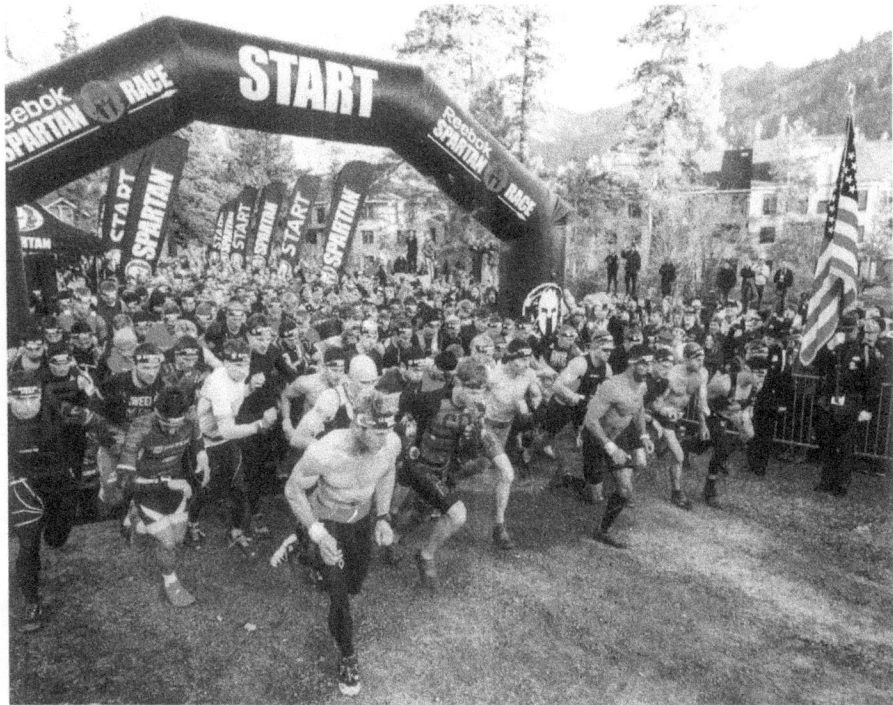

Elite male athletes at the start of the 2017 " Spartan World Championship" in North Lake Tahoe, CA. The race featured athletes from more than fifty countries.

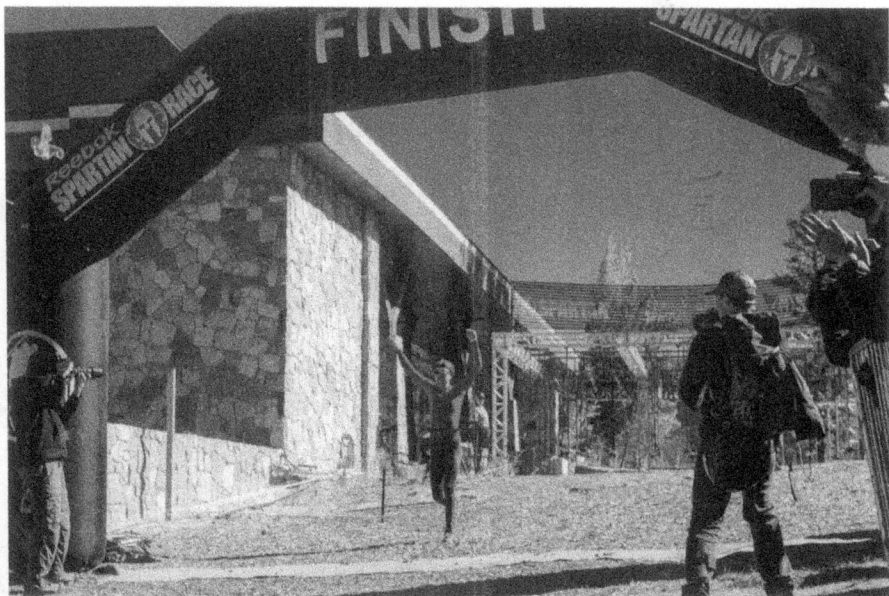

The Czech Republic's Zuzana Kocumová crossing the finish line to win the 2016 Spartan World Championship in North Lake Tahoe, CA. The race featured athletes from more than thirty countries.

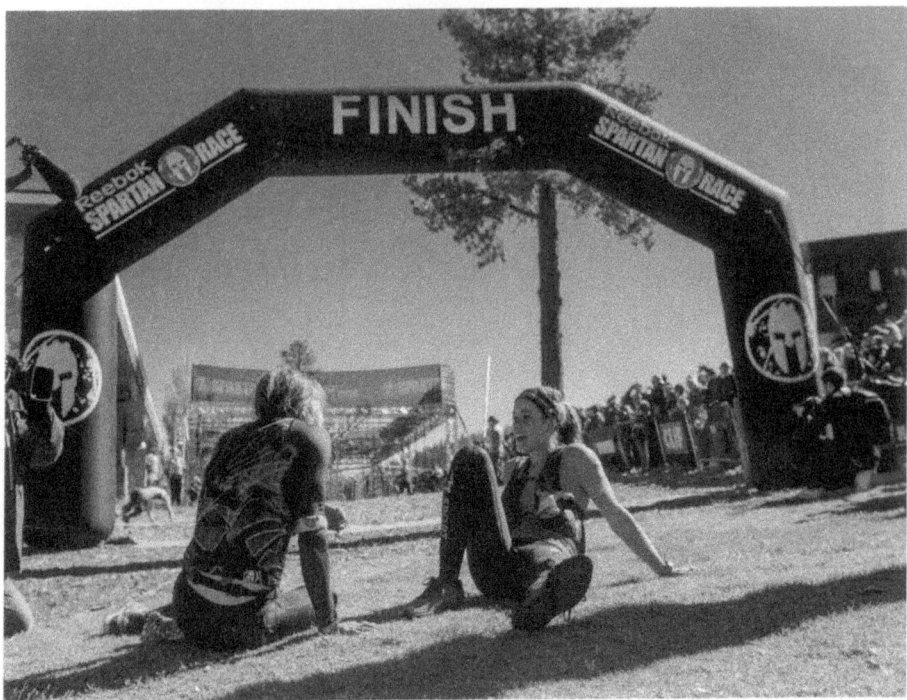

Athletes Faye Stennning (left) and Lindsay Webster (right) catching up after a photo finish at the 2016 Spartan World Championship. Webster placed second, milliseconds ahead of Stenning who finished third.

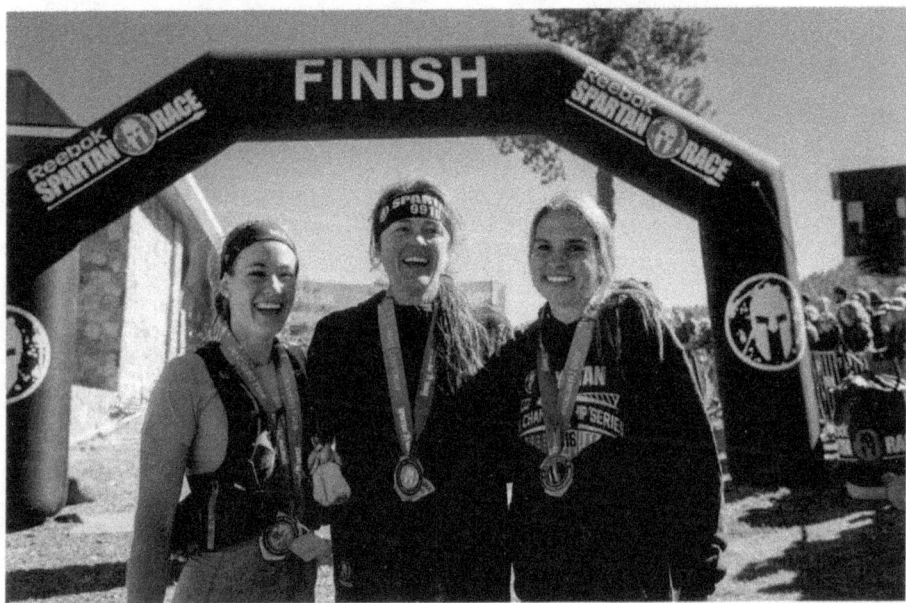

The Czech Republic's Zuzana Kocumová after winning the 2016 Spartan World Championship in North Lake Tahoe, CA. The race featured athletes from more than thirty countries.

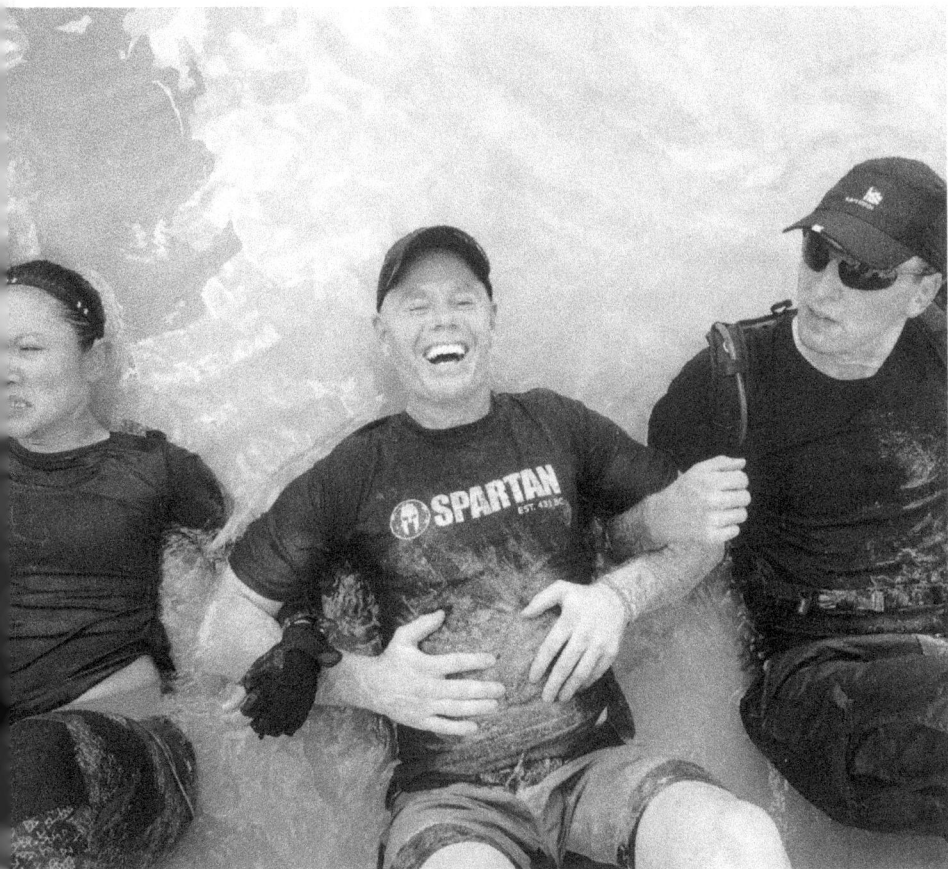

...n dragging participants through the mud during the 2016 Hurricane Heat in Bintan Island, ...donesia.

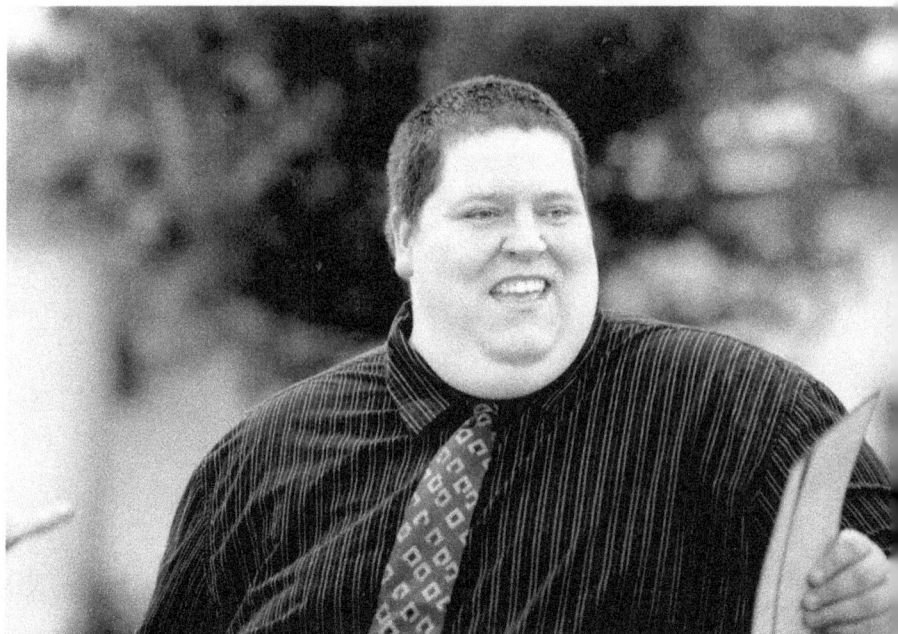

This is Chris Davis weighing in at 696 pounds, before we helped him drop down to 262 pounds to r
his first Spartan Ultra Beast in 2012.

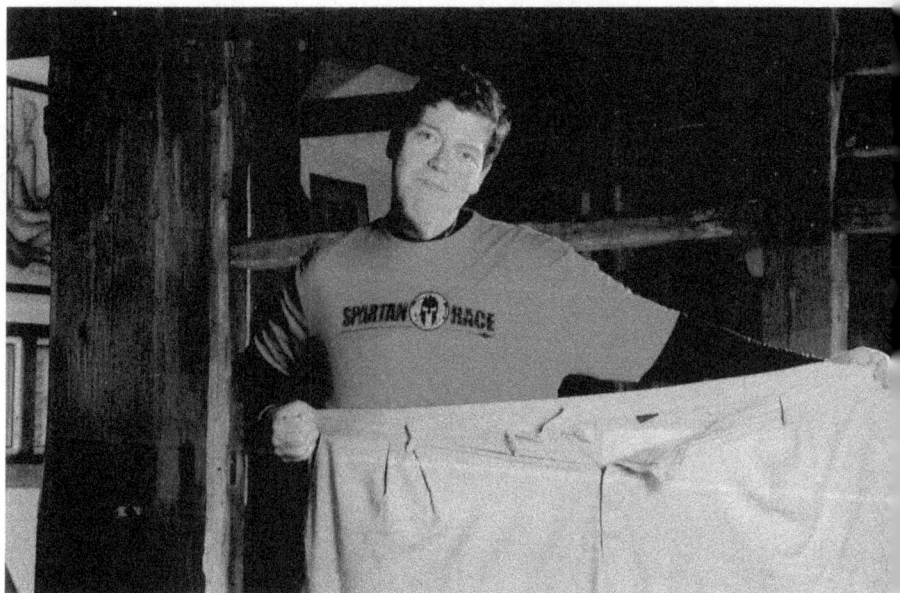

This is Chris Davis in my barn on Riverside Farm in Vermont, showing off the pants he wore when
weighed 696 pounds.

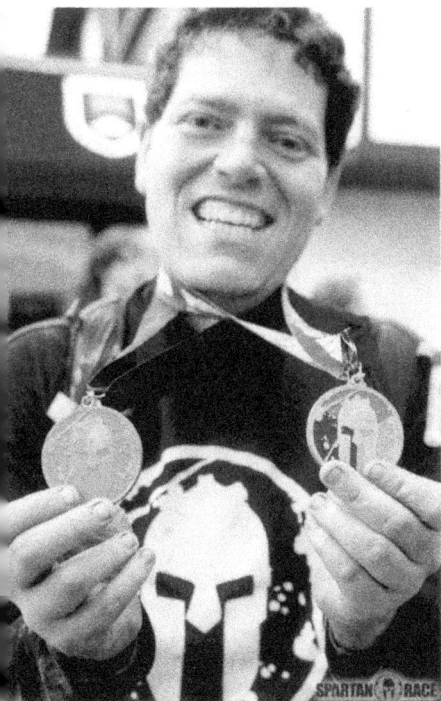

Here's Chris Davis weighing in at 262 pounds after finishing the Spartan Ultra Beast in Killington, VT, in 2012.

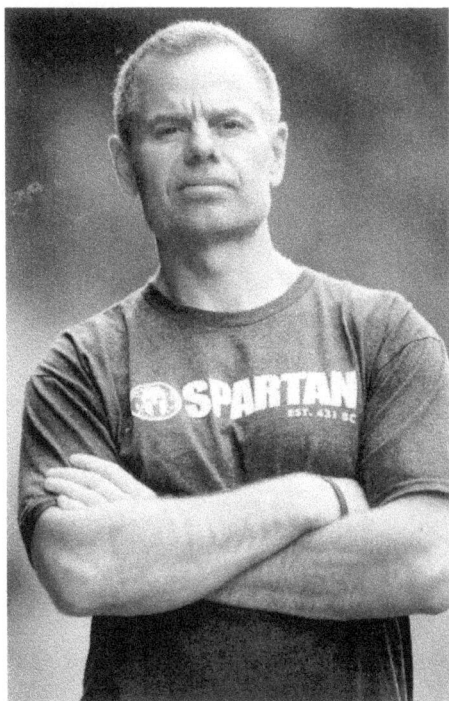

Joe De Sena

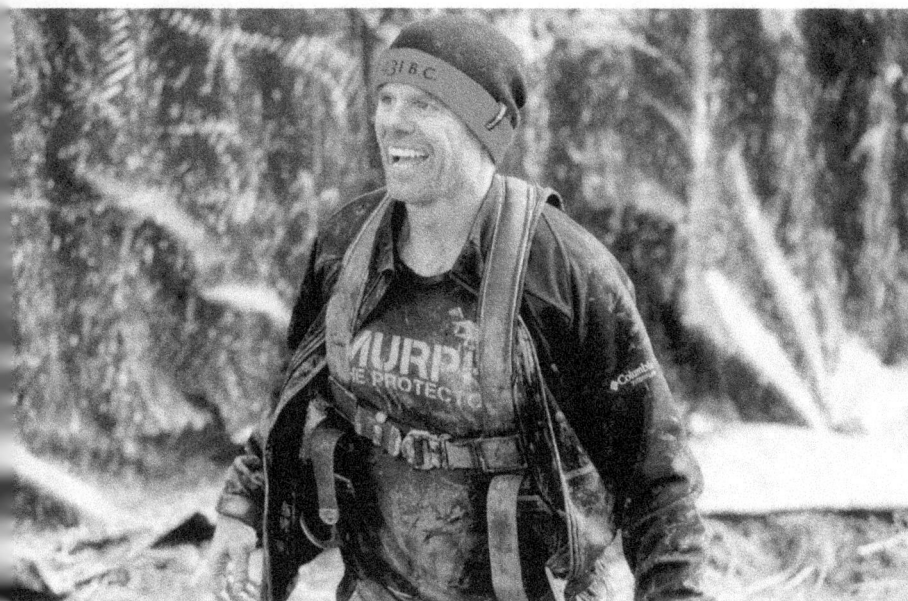

This is me at the Ohio Super in 2014. I completed that race in a wheelchair after been challenged by Michael Mills, the first wheelchair-bound man to complete a Spartan event.

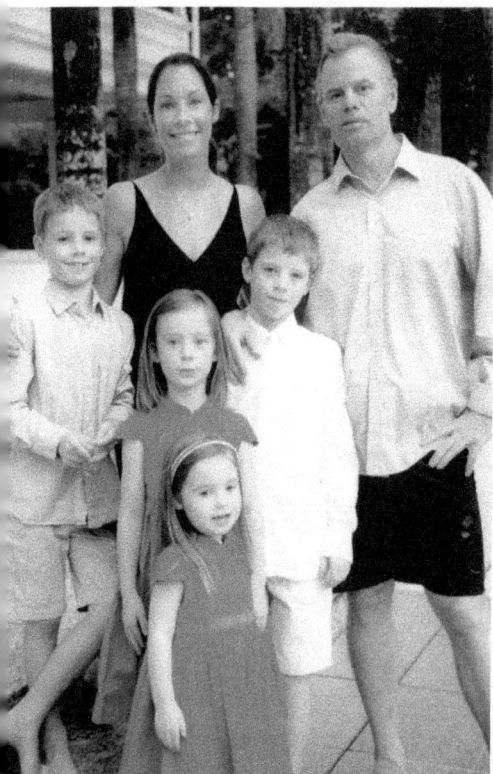

This is my family during the holidays in Singapore in 2015. That's my wife, Courtney, with our kids Jack (back left), Charlie (back right), Katherine (middle), and Alexandra (front).

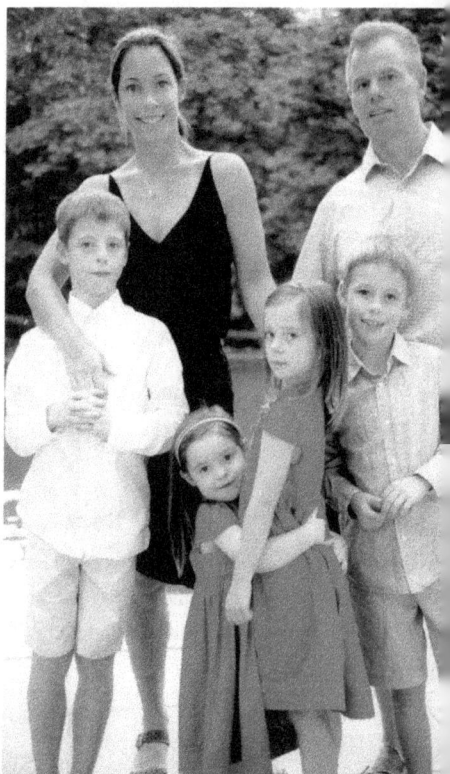

This is my family during the holidays in Singapore in 2015. That's my wife, Courtney, with our kids (left to right) Jack, Alexandra, Katherine, Charlie.

Angela Duckworth tells me Spartan is on the right track. "If it's true that gritty people are not insane, that in fact what they have is hope, then experiences that show you that there is hope in things you thought were difficult or not possible, could generalize across all your life."

Suddenly you realize that the marriage that's floundering, the job you hate, the business idea you can't seem to get off the ground can be examined under a new light. You can find yourself grittier than you ever thought you could be. Your life isn't a walk-on part in someone else's headliner. Your life is all yours. What you do with it now is up to you.

GET OFF THE COUCH!
How to Get Gritty

Step 1. MEMORIZE THE FORMULA FOR GRIT.

Passion + Persistence + Time = GRIT.

Step 2. SCORE YOUR GRIT LEVEL. Take the Courage Test below. Choose one response from each of the following twelve statements about yourself. There are no right or wrong answers. Be honest to generate the most accurate score.

THE GRIT TEST
HOW GRITTY ARE YOU?

1. I have overcome setbacks to conquer an important challenge.
   - Very much like me
   - Mostly like me
   - Somewhat like me
   - Not much like me
   - Not like me at all

2. New ideas and projects sometimes distract me from previous ones.
   - ○ Very much like me
   - ○ Mostly like me
   - ○ Somewhat like me
   - ○ Not much like me
   - ○ Not like me at all

3. My interests change from year to year.
   - ○ Very much like me
   - ○ Mostly like me
   - ○ Somewhat like me
   - ○ Not much like me
   - ○ Not like me at all

4. Setbacks don't discourage me.
   - ○ Very much like me
   - ○ Mostly like me
   - ○ Somewhat like me
   - ○ Not much like me
   - ○ Not like me at all

5. I have been obsessed with a certain idea or project for a short time but later lost interest.
   - ○ Very much like me
   - ○ Mostly like me
   - ○ Somewhat like me
   - ○ Not much like me
   - ○ Not like me at all

6. I am a hard worker.
   - ○ Very much like me
   - ○ Mostly like me
   - ○ Somewhat like me
   - ○ Not much like me
   - ○ Not like me at all

7. I often set a goal but later choose to pursue a different one.
   - ○ Very much like me
   - ○ Mostly like me
   - ○ Somewhat like me
   - ○ Not much like me
   - ○ Not like me at all

8. I have difficulty maintaining my focus on projects that take more than a few months to complete.
   - ○ Very much like me
   - ○ Mostly like me
   - ○ Somewhat like me
   - ○ Not much like me
   - ○ Not like me at all

9. I finish whatever I begin.
   - ○ Very much like me
   - ○ Mostly like me
   - ○ Somewhat like me
   - ○ Not much like me
   - ○ Not like me at all

10. I have achieved a goal that took years of work.
   - ○ Very much like me
   - ○ Mostly like me
   - ○ Somewhat like me
   - ○ Not much like me
   - ○ Not like me at all

11. I become interested in new pursuits every few months.
   - ○ Very much like me
   - ○ Mostly like me
   - ○ Somewhat like me
   - ○ Not much like me
   - ○ Not like me at all

12. I am diligent.
   - ○ Very much like me
   - ○ Mostly like me
   - ○ Somewhat like me
   - ○ Not much like me
   - ○ Not like me at all

SCORING:

1. For questions 1, 4, 6, 9, 10 and 12 assign the following points:
   - 5 = Very much like me
   - 4 = Mostly like me
   - 3 = Somewhat like me
   - 2 = Not much like me
   - 1 = Not like me at all

2. For questions 2, 3, 5, 7, 8 and 11 assign the following points:
- 1 = Very much like me
- 2 = Mostly like me
- 3 = Somewhat like me
- 4 = Not much like me
- 5 = Not like me at all

Add up all the points and divide by 12. The maximum score on this scale is 5 (extremely gritty), and the lowest scale on this scale is 1 (not at all gritty).

Record your Grit level here _____

Extracted from Duckworth, A.L., Peterson, C., Matthews, M.D., and Kelly, D.R. (2007). Grit: Perseverance and passion for long-term goals. *Journal of Personality and Social Psychology, 9,* 1087–1101.

Step 3. GET GRITTIER. Go back to Principle #1: Find Your True North. Write down your goal and brainstorm all the ways you can level up your grit in every aspect of your life to reach that dream:

ACTION STEPS TO 10X MY GRIT

At Home _____

At Work_____

In My Relationships_____

In Time Management_____

In My Health and Fitness_____

PRINCIPLE #7

EMBRACE ADVERSITY

Fire is the test of gold, adversity of strong men.
—SENECA THE YOUNGER

Unless a man has been kicked around a little, you can't really
depend upon him to amount to anything.
—WILLIAM FEATHER

A wounded deer leaps the highest.
—EMILY DICKENSON

Most of us have things way too easy. We face very little adversity in our lives. And that's a shame because adversity builds character. That's why I like to manufacture adversity. A Spartan Race is manufactured adversity. The obstacles are designed to be really tough to show people that they can overcome adversity and find growth in the accomplishment.

I carry a forty-six-pound kettlebell with me wherever I go to manu-facture some adversity into my daily life. It reminds me how good I have it. People look at me as if I'm a little crazy, but it's better than the sandbag I used to carry. I don't have to explain myself so often; after all, a kettle-bell has a handle.

Women everywhere are going to hate me when I tell this story: When Courtney went into labor with our first child on our way to the hospital, I parked about a mile away and made us walk. We even climbed the stairs to the delivery room instead of taking a wheelchair and using the elevator. Hey, a lot of women in many other cultures walked much far-ther and faced much greater adversity to deliver babies. Courtney was strong. I knew she could do it. And when we got to delivery, the baby came right out.

The adversities we have faced pale in comparison to those that some people have endured. I'm fascinated by the stories of people who have sur-vived enormous hardship and have been transformed as a result. One of the most compelling I've heard comes from Karim Jaude, a Lebanese-born real estate investor now living in the United States.

In 1979, Karim was sitting in the restaurant of the Hilton Hotel in downtown Tehran when he received a phone call: "Don't come home," the voice on the end of the phone whispered. "We have *visitors*." Then the line went dead. Karim gently replaced the receiver in its cradle.

"Please, put on the television," he asked a passing waiter.

The atmosphere in the city had been tense for several months. His friend, the leader of the former ruling family of Iran, Shah Pahlavi, had left the country for exile in Egypt earlier that year. Since his departure, Iran was becoming more and more unstable. The Ayatollah Khomeini's pro-visional revolutionary government was growing in power.

In the corner of the restaurant, the television set showed images of dem-onstrators marching through the streets. Windows were being smashed, stores looted. In some parts of the city, gangs had begun to gather. Armed guerrilla fighters shot at soldiers. The restaurant went silent as the diners turned at their tables and watched the screen in horror.

Karim knew he couldn't go home. He would find out later that three armed men had forced their way in to his house and ransacked it. What they didn't take with them they smashed or shredded, including a small Picasso painting he had bought on a business trip to London. As a wealthy young man, much indebted to the Shah for helping him rebuild his life at a pivotal moment, Karim was now a target.

He left the restaurant to roam the streets and figure out a plan. What would he do? Where could he go? Fires burned on street corners, shattered glass was everywhere. Karim decided he had no choice but to go to the Lebanese embassy.

It was not the best solution. He had escaped from Lebanon three years earlier after being kidnapped and tortured by Syrian militants. His home country was in turmoil, and now, it seemed, his adopted country of Iran was beginning to feel the same way. As he headed toward the Lebanese embassy, Karim thought about what had happened to him during his thirty-eight years.

He'd had an idyllic childhood in Beirut, the Paris of the East, watching his father, uncles, and brothers build a thriving construction business. He started his own career in real estate at age fifteen. Ten years later, he would make his first million, and by the time he was thirty-five years old he employed 1,265 people.

Then, Beirut changed. Syrian warmongers spilled over the borders and Karim was targeted for his business successes and political ties. Once, he was stopped on the street in Beirut and thrown into the back of a van. He was interrogated seven times and tortured, hung upside down, and whipped until he bled. His kidnappers gave him electric shocks. They

MASTER CLASS
Mark Webb, Death Racer, amputee

Mark Webb, a single father and regular Spartan Death Racer, recently lost part of his left leg in a motorcycle accident. In an interview shortly after his surgery, he said his big motivator is his son; he wants to show his son that setbacks in life can be the fuel that propels greater drive. Here, Mark discusses how to keep going when your mind doesn't want to.

FINDING MOTIVATION

I've had days when I just don't want to move. I don't have the energy. On days like that sometimes you just need to give yourself a little push. Plan to chip away at 20 percent of what you planned to do. Don't do the eight-mile run, do the two-mile. Just do something. And more often than not that'll put you right back on track. The key to consistency—and a much more critical component than motivation—is momentum. Once you apply the energy to get started, it is relatively easy to keep going. The "mind trick" that I use to continue to push myself physically, at work, or in anything I attempt to achieve, is that getting started is the most important step because it provides the basis for momentum.

kicked him in the stomach and demanded he hand over his wealth. He thought he was going to die.

Luckily, he negotiated his release but was told to leave Lebanon forever. He ended up in Iran where some friends helped him start a new life. But now, here he was, walking toward the Lebanese embassy in Tehran, once again down to nothing.

The building was deserted. The gates were chained. He needed a plan B. Karim knew he had to leave the country. And with the roads and airports closed, he would have to take his chances by train.

When Khomeini came to power, he ordered every woman over the age of ten to wear a *chador,* a black robe covering the body from head to toe and niqab with a slit for the eyes. Karim found a store and quickly bought one. Hiding himself under the heavy black cloth, he boarded a train. Over the next fourteen days, Karim traveled by train, bus, mule, bicycle, and on foot to Bahrain. There, a friend put him on a flight to Paris and then to the United States. He arrived at LAX with $17 in his pocket.

Few people could have endured what Karim went through. Twice, he had the success he had built taken from him under brutal circumstances. But he didn't give up. Los Angeles was just another beginning. When I met him a couple of years ago and he told me his incredible tale, he had been living in L.A. for nearly thirty years. During that time, he had created a multimillion-dollar real estate business that continues to thrive today.

It's hard to hear a story like Karim's and not be affected. It had great impact on me. I had never experienced such hardship. When I asked Karim what had enabled him to move past these events, he blew me away with another story about something his father taught him.

When he was very young, his father had an accident that left him bedridden. One day, just after World War II had ended, Karim asked his father, "Dad, you said the war is over. How come there are still innocent people being killed?" Karim was seventy when he recounted the story to me. "My father hugged me and told me, 'In the history of man, there has never been justice in the world, and there will never *ever* be. But what you and I can do is to help reduce other people's suffering and not add to it.'"

This principle became the driving force behind Karim's life.

The positive impact he could have on others motivated him to make money. At the age of twenty-six when he made his first million, he started a foundation to help poor children go to school. His own education had been hard won, and he didn't want other kids in his home country to suffer the same hardship. Following that, he started a second foundation, aiding people who couldn't afford medical care. He founded it in memory of his father who had passed away because he couldn't get the necessary help to rehabilitate himself after his accident. "In truth for the last forty years, my religion has been to help at least one person a day," Karim said, "and it has never failed."

This has been his True North, helping to direct him down one steady path. This ideal also enabled him to judge the choices he had to make in life. He has used the most adverse experiences of his life not just to push himself on, but to remind himself of his good fortune. "Some of my friends who were kidnapped killed themselves afterward," he told me. "So that means I have two choices. I can sit in a corner and whine or I can go on with my life. I chose to go on."

Karim's extraordinary hardships are something few of us in the Western world ever face. But still, we all have our own tough luck and challenges to endure. I like to say that obstacles have everyone's address. Yet some people suck it up and bounce back while others fall apart.

Aristotle called courage the first virtue, because it makes all of the other virtues possible. It helps us become more self-aware; it fuels our passion and our grit. Those who are courageous are better able at dealing with life's curveballs. But where does the ability to act with courage come from?

When I hear stories of people like Karim, I wonder if their hardships fueled their successes. There are many examples: Take Ben Franklin, for example. His parents could afford to keep him in school only until his tenth birthday. Even though he was forced to drop out of school at this young age, he still studied on his own and became an inventor and one of the most accomplished of America's Founding Fathers.

Franklin Roosevelt became partially paralyzed at age thirty-nine after developing polio. His confinement to a wheelchair didn't prevent him from going on to lead the country as one of the most popular presidents of all time. Surfer Bethany Hamilton survived a shark attack at age thirteen and lost her left arm in the accident. This didn't stop her from becoming a professional surfer and an inspiration to millions. "I don't need easy," Bethany has said. "I just need possible." These are just some stories of well-known people who have overcome adversity to build hugely successful lives. There are millions more stories like theirs all around us. Were these people naturally resilient, or was their resilience a byproduct of enduring adversity?

This was something that developmental psychologists Emmy Werner and Ruth Smith wanted to know, too. Their longitudinal study is the only one to date to track if and how resilience can be built up in people exposed to any kind of adversity, from the time they were in the womb through middle age. Beginning in 1955, they followed 698 children born that same year on the Hawaiian island of Kauai.

As it turned out, about a third of the kids they followed had been born into extremely adverse situations: families struggling with abject poverty, alcoholism, and mental illness. Many of these kids had developed serious learning and behavior problems by the age of ten. But here's the surprise: When Werner and Smith published their findings five decades later, they were able to show that not all of the kids growing up at risk reacted to their stressors in the same way. In fact, one-third of the kids that the two psychologists ended up calling "vulnerable, but invincible," displayed all the hallmarks of successful living. They didn't just excel in school, they often exceeded those children who had grown up in more economically secure and stable homes. They grew into adults with good lives. None of them ever relied on social services or got into trouble with the law. They even had much lower rates of divorce and fewer chronic health problems by age forty than the more fortunate kids turned out to have. Werner and Smith wrote, "Their very existence challenges the myth that a child who is a member of a so-called 'high-risk' group is fated to become one of life's losers."

Werner and Smith identified three key elements that buffered the kids against life's cruel blows.

The first was an internal one: The kids were nice. Even as babies they were friendly and good-natured. They were good at figuring things out on their own. As they grew, these traits developed into helpfulness and confidence.

The second factor: These kids forged a strong bond with at least one functioning family member. This could be a parent or someone from their extended family like a grandparent. The psychologists said that the resilient children seemed good at recruiting surrogate parents. That was true of Karim Jaude. When his father died, Karim turned to his uncles.

The third protective factor that made a difference was community support, usually a coach or favorite teacher. What's interesting is that when these kids became successful adults, they continued to seek out community mentors when they needed help.

So how does all this reflect on your journey to be a Spartan? Well, I think you'll get the most out of embracing adversity when you recruit people to help you overcome it. Have a look at the people around you. You'll succeed more if you have people to depend on. People you've made a commitment to and people who are committed to you. Seek out mentors. Can't find any? Look harder. Extend yourself.

And embrace adversity. Don't run from it. Reframe your attitude toward it: Adversity is the surest path to success when you attack it. Every day, you are going to face hardship, and some of your suffering is going to be extreme, so you had better get good practice dealing with it.

I like what Dennis Charney has to say in his book *Resilience: The Science of Mastering Life's Greatest Challenges*. Dr. Charney has spent years studying war veterans and victims of psychological and physical abuse. He says they've told him the secret to mustering the courage to overcome new obstacles is to replay in their minds the times when they crushed similar obstacles. Knowing you've attacked adversity once prepares you to attack it again. The more you attack, the more you're *able* to attack.

As I mentioned before, one of the reasons my wife and I move our family to live in other countries is to embrace adversity by forcing ourselves out of our comfort zone. Our family is great and rolls with the punches. They are like Bruce Lee: They are taking the good they learn and discarding the not so useful. It's a very hard thing to do because you leave lots of *connections*—friends and family—and comfort behind, but it is a unique educational experience!

I call deliberately stepping into adverse situations purposeful suffering, and you can train for it. Behavioral scientists call it "stress inoculation." You make yourself immune to stress by exposing yourself to whatever it is you fear over and over again. It's really just moving outside your comfort zone on a daily basis. And the Spartans? Well, they just call it life.

GET OFF THE COUCH!
How to Embrace Adversity

Step 1. GET BUSY. Remember back when you were taking the SATs or some other timed test? Did this ever happen to you? When the proctor announced, "Five minutes left," you panicked, started worrying about how many questions you'd left unanswered, and became paralyzed with fear and anxiety. When your emotions take over, the best strategy is to get your body and hands moving. Do the work. Force yourself to get out of your head and on to solving the problems at hand.

Resilient people know that action is the antidote to anxiety. Quell your emotions by getting busy, being productive. This is something you can practice by putting yourself into situations of "deliberate adversity." During training, astronauts, Navy SEALs, police officers, and firefighters are routinely placed in challenging scenarios with unknown variables to exercise their ability to take quick action and take control of the situation using a cool head. It's a survival skill. And the more times they practice being resourceful and resilient in an adverse situation, the more confident they become in their ability to deal with any surprise. Remember my kayak combat roll example? You can practice all the Eskimo rolls you want in the calm waters of a swimming pool or lake, but until you practice combat rolls in your kayak in the middle of raging Class IV rapids, you'll never know if you can roll when it's really necessary.

Step 2. LEARN TO BREATHE. When you are in a stressful situation (facing adversity), your breathing tends to quicken and you take shallow breaths because your body feels like it's not getting enough oxygen. But hyperventilation actually makes anxiety worse and can trigger chest pains, weakness, and rapid heartbeat. It can make you feel faint. All of this will make it more difficult to deal effectively with the adversity that is causing your stress to begin with. Think about the benefits of being able to diffuse anxious, shallow breathing quickly when you need to in an adverse environment. And take note of how the real pros do it.

The biathlon event in the Winter Olympics combines cross-country skiing and target shooting with a 22-caliber rifle. Churning his legs and arms to get swiftly across rugged alpine terrain, a biathlete's heart rate hits two hundred beats per minute. Then he must stop, un-sling his rifle, and bring his heart rate down enough to steady his hands and mind to take aim at a target fifty meters away. A top biathlete can lower his heart rate to 140 beats per minute in just twenty seconds in order to be calm and steady enough to aim accurately. How? By training his body through deep breathing techniques and by exhaling extra CO_2 to counteract the lactic acid buildup in his muscles. You can use the same technique when in the throes of panic and faced with a trauma or anxiety-producing adversity. Try it now:

Do fifteen burpees to simulate the rapid, shallow breathing of a panic attack. Next, blow out with a strong, deliberate abdominal contraction by pulling your belly button back toward your spine. This forces a higher volume-in breath. Now, relax your belly and breathe in deeply, allowing your belly to rise before your chest to ensure that you fill your entire lung space. Bringing a higher volume of oxygen into your lungs will relax you by stimulating the parasympathetic nervous system. Do it again and again as you feel your heart rate start to return to normal. When you're relaxed with a head full of oxygenated blood in your brain, you are better able to focus and devise a solution out of the adversity you're facing.

Step 3. EMBRACE ADVERSITY AND EXPERIENCE IT OFTEN. By repeatedly experiencing hardship and pain, you build tolerance and readiness for when adversity comes again. And it will come again and again. Exercise: Identify the adversity in your life in the following categories. Write down the details of each struggle.

Adversity at Work

_____

_____

_____

Adversity at Home

_____

_____

_____

Adversity in Relationships

_____

_____

_____

Adversity in Health or Fitness

_____

_____

_____

Step 4. DEVELOP STRATEGIES TO OVERCOME ADVERSITY. As you get more practice dealing with adverse situations, you'll find certain strategies that work for you. Here are some techniques Spartans use effectively. Try them. Adapt them. Make them your own.

>> Keep your focus on your True North. Don't compromise.

>> Commit to your passion. Make a pledge or unwavering promise to yourself.

>> Ask yourself, "What's the upside and downside of taking a certain action?"

>> Get busy. Always move forward through your adversity.

>> Grit it out. Never quit.

ADJUST YOUR FRAME OF REFERENCE

If we were logical, the future would be bleak indeed. But we are more than logical.
We are human beings, and we have faith, and we have hope, and we can work.

—JACQUES COUSTEAU

Optimism is the faith that leads to achievement.

—HELEN KELLER

One morning when I was on a ski trip in northern Japan, I woke up and couldn't see. Everything was blurry. I couldn't make anything out. I figured I was dehydrated and needed some sugar, so I had some water and an orange. Nothing changed. I was still stumbling around and bumping into things. I thought, "This has to be fixable," so I took a cold shower. Still blind. My wife rushed me to the hospital.

No one at the hospital spoke English. One doctor jumped into motion. He took an MRI machine and quickly determined that I had a blood clot in my brain, which was affecting nerves controlling my eyes. They started me on blood thinners. I was laying there attached to all these wires and tubes, and thinking, "This may be the last time I ski with my kids."

I was in darkness at a tiny hospital in the middle of nowhere, the doctors didn't speak English, and I didn't speak Japanese. I was scared. They say a healthy person has a thousand wishes but a sick person has only one wish—to get well. Ironically, not being able to see opened my eyes to what was important in life—being healthy. It changed my frame of reference.

The next day I went from being completely upset to saying, "Okay, what's my plan here? I have to change my frame of reference. No more feeling worried and frustrated. I have to do something."

I figured that I had to get blood flow to my head. Maybe that would help. So I started doing burpees, mobility exercises, and upside-down push-ups. I put my head in a bowl of ice water. The doctors looked at me like, "Who is this crazy American doing exercises and taking cold showers?"

Then a young doctor who spoke a little English passed through and took an interest in my case. She was visiting from a larger hospital four hours away and she arranged to transfer me there. I stayed for the next twenty-five days. She ran all sorts of tests on me. In the end, it turned out that I, like 20 percent of the world's population, have a tiny hole in my heart less than a millimeter in diameter. That's what triggered the blood clot that made its way to my brain.

Finally after thirty days on blood thinners and burpees, I got my eyesight back. The experience gave me a whole new appreciation for my sight, my health, and just how lucky I've been. God was just toying with me, with this minor glitch in Japan.

Many people have faced much, much worse. If you're ever feeling defeated and want to change your frame of reference, visit Walter Reed National Military Medical Center. That's where you'll witness real adversity and grit in the veterans rehabbing from terrible injuries.

I saw some of these men and women at the opening of a handicap-accessible house near Poplar Grove, Illinois. The facility was funded by the Oscar Mike Foundation (oscarmike.org), which is involved with Spartan. It's a place for injured vets to stay and bond while they attend sports clinics designed to help them understand that there's the hope of living a healthy, athletic life after injury.

This house is a great place filled with amazing people. I took my nine-year-old daughter to the opening because I wanted her to meet some people who have extreme challenges in their lives. People like Noah Currier, the founder of Oscar Mike.

Oscar Mike takes its name from the military radio term meaning "On the Move." The foundation has a lifestyle apparel brand that funnels all sales proceeds and donations into a program to help rehabilitate injured veterans through adaptive sports events. Noah and a few other injured vets started it on Veteran's Day in 2011.

"Adaptive sports literally saved me and I knew I had to share that with others," Noah said as he moved into his story. He was a Marine corporal, one of the first to be deployed to Afghanistan after the September 11 attacks, and he also served in Iraq in 2003. After seven months in Iraq, he returned to Camp Pendleton. A few days later, he was in a car when a fellow Marine fell asleep at the wheel. They crashed down an embankment. The accident left Noah paralyzed from the chest down. Shortly after he finished rehab, he came home. Just days later, his girlfriend fell asleep while driving and was killed.

"Losing her was the nail in the coffin for me. I had nothing to live for," he told me. Noah was in a funk for about six years, drinking, doing drugs. A buddy of his knew he was in a bad place and tried to help. After a lot of

MASTER CLASS
Christian Banda, Spartan Racer, 34

In the summer of 2014, my doctor told me I had Parkinson's disease. For several years before this, my right hand twitched and then the twitching moved to my right foot. I had a special brain scan that confirmed the diagnosis.

I was thirty-four.

Becoming symptomatic at such a young age is nearly unheard of, my doctor said. Then she handed me a prescription.

The most visible PD symptom is a tremor followed by slow movements, muscle stiffness, and postural instability. The disease literally robs you of your ability to move. It impairs your fine and gross motor skills and, eventually, your ability to speak. Some secondary symptoms include anxiety, depression, loss of smell, sleep disturbances, cognitive issues such as slow thinking, and memory difficulties. There are many more.

I grew incredibly depressed. The news of Robin Williams having PD and Lewy body dementia hit me hard. I kept thinking, "Stop shaking! I can control this!" If you had a conversation with me during that time, I was only able to comprehend every third word you said. My wife did not know what to do.

A friend recommended I see a movement disorders specialist, and soon I was in the care of one of the top Parkinson's doctors in the country. He changed my dosages. He spent almost two hours explaining Parkinson's and its treatments and assured me that I would be able to live a full life with PD. He also said that *exercise* would be essential in slowing the progression of the disease.

I began exercising. Up to this point, I hadn't done much, just two 5K races.

My wife signed us up for a Spartan Race. And it changed my life.

I thought Spartan was a 5K, so I trained for one. But she signed us up for a Spartan Super, an eight-plus-mile obstacle course. I was terrified. I was not fit enough. I was in complete agony from the beginning.

My life changed at an eight-foot wall obstacle. I grabbed the top of it, smashed my foot, and fell. A fellow Spartan asked if I was okay. I said I had Parkinson's. It was the first time I ever told anyone outside of my circle of trust.

The guy helped me over the wall.

For the next five miles, I limped and hobbled through obstacles thinking of my family and what they mean to me. That wall encounter with the stranger changed my perception of my disease. It sparked something in me that would become a roaring blaze. That day, I became a warrior in the battle against Parkinson's.

Today, I eat healthy and I train like an elite athlete. I am a trail runner, which helps my balance and stability. I lift weights to have better control of my body. I'm down to 165 pounds. I have finished five Spartan races, becoming the first person with Parkinson's to complete a Spartan Trifecta.

My wife is my personal trainer and runs every race by my side. I have seen her cry at races when my legs do not want to work with my body. Her love for me motivates me to push harder.

I once viewed my condition as a death sentence. Now, I look at it as if I was chosen to do great things. I realize that Parkinson's is a part of me, but it does not define me. Instead, I now see how it has elevated me to another level of grit, determination, and perseverance that has strengthened me in all aspects of my life.

begging and pleading, he took Noah to Aspen, Colorado, to ski down a mountain with an instructor.

"I didn't think it was possible," Noah said. "Then I'm at the top of Snowmass Mountain, twelve thousand feet. You're above the clouds. It feels like you can see forever. When all you know up to this point is your bedroom in your parent's house or the side of a bar, and you see this, it's a religious experience. It changed my frame of reference. I realized there was a whole new world out there ahead of me."

Noah made it down the mountain. "That was the best time of my life," he said. "The sky's the limit. Let's go skydiving. Let's go surfing."

He went to college and "became addicted" to competitive sports. He's involved in weight lifting, rowing, skiing, and hand cycling. At a competition, he and a group of athletes were brainstorming ways to get more injured vets involved and Oscar Mike was born.

"Once you start getting physically active again, you get a piece of you back," Noah explained. "That adrenaline comes back and you start living the way you used to live. So we wanted to help our brothers and sisters embrace that Oscar Mike mentality and get back on the move. Injured soldiers aren't looking for handouts; they want the ability to take charge of their own lives."

We've had injured vets come out to compete in Spartan Races. You'll have twenty people helping a paralyzed vet through the course obstacles. I'm sure that vet finishes the course a different person. And I have to believe that some of the five thousand Spartans who pass by him or her on their way through the course change their frame of reference, too.

Seeing someone else struggle with hardship can make you look at your life differently, like when you realize your tolerance for discomfort is so low that you flip out if the bus breaks down and have to walk an extra block to work. A life spent looking for the easy way lessens our faith in our own abilities. It becomes too easy to feel victimized when things get tough. The way to avoid that mess is to recognize it and then adjust your frame of reference.

We all build assumptions and attitudes that shape how we see the world. We use this frame of reference to make decisions and judgments. A frame of reference is a useful tool most of the time. But if you never change it or look beyond the frame, you can miss out on life-changing options. Look at Noah. The summit of that mountain gave him the perspective to see the possibilities at the bottom of that ski slope. Adjusting your frame of reference can reveal the hidden path through life's minefields. It's a critical skill to learn to get to your True North.

One year when I was working on my pool business in Howard Beach, New York, I hired some Eastern European workers. This was back in the late eighties, and a lot of them had left their countries during the fall of communist rule. I couldn't believe how hard those guys worked. They were first to arrive and the last to leave the jobsite. They did most of the work, and I never heard a complaint. I could barely keep up with them. Then I realized that the living and working conditions that they had left were so much tougher than they were here in the United States. This pool business was easy compared to what they were used to, and they appreciated the work. In other words, their idea of tough work came from an entirely different frame of reference than mine.

The Greek philosophers known as the Stoics knew the value of changing the frame of reference. The Stoics embraced hardship and poverty. One of the best-known Stoics, Seneca the Younger, was very wealthy but he would "practice poverty." He believed the wealthy should experience being poor by wearing shabby clothes and scavenging for food. He wrote, "A man's as miserable as he thinks he is." By regularly rehearsing being poor, he rationalized, your perception of your current situation would radically change so that you'd come to appreciate what you already had.

WHAT I'VE LEARNED
Dick Costolo, former CEO of Twitter

Rely on your team. [The Spartan course] is a physical manifestation of why teamwork allows you to be more successful than the guy out there doing it himself. The coolest thing I saw out there were the obstacles that you really needed to work with somebody to get over. Sure, you could grind through it yourself and probably make it, but if you worked with a team you'd get through it faster—those things are awesome team-building exercises.

Try changing how you think. Hate your small apartment? Live in a tent for a week, and you'll learn to be grateful for the four walls of your home. Dying to go to that pricy new restaurant in town? Fast for three days and you'll be delighted with a simple apple or can of tuna fish. Frustrated by the crowded bus? Start walking to work, and I bet you'll appreciate public transportation pretty quickly.

What you're doing is practicing self-imposed adversity. By deliberately putting yourself in tough situations you see what you can endure. You question your current assumptions about yourself and your life. Try changing your frame of reference and you'll see the breadth of options you have and realize anything is possible.

In the 1960s, a Polish psychiatrist named Kazimierz Dąbrowski formed a fascinating theory related to all this. Dabrowski had seen horrors on the battlefield in World War I and been imprisoned by both the Nazis in World War II and the communists in postwar Poland. He was interested in personality development and was curious to know what enabled some people to behave heroically and others brutally.

He came up with the idea that adverse emotions like fear, anxiety, and frustration were necessary to becoming a psychologically strong person. Dabrowski believed that most people live their lives influenced by their biological impulses and by pandering to peer pressure. They face a lot of external conflict as they battle others to "get their way" or be "paid their dues."

Occasionally, though, a person faces a life hurdle that changes everything. Suddenly, they start to reflect on their values and actions. They are forced to reconsider the automatic associations they've always made before. The adversity they're facing is challenging their viewpoint and changing their behavior. It's changing their vision of how life ought to be.

A Spartan SGX coach named Rich Borgatti had one of these experiences on Killington Mountain, Vermont, during the 2014 Spartan World Championship Beast.

"I had a choice on the mountain," he says. "I could let it beat me, or I could smile and say I chose to be there, even though it was a grueling eight hours. After the race, I came home, and nothing was really that hard anymore. My kids, my business—I just had a sense of peace that I didn't have before."

That is what I mean by changing your frame of reference. It's responding to a struggle that causes a change in your attitude. It can happen on a small scale. You can start taking cold showers, which reminds you that having to walk home in the rain is no biggie. You can do one hundred burpees every day and realize that yanking a tree stump out of the yard is a piece of cake. Doing little things can have a big effect. Here's an example: Michael Phelps's coach used to occasionally crack his swim goggles in training so that they'd fill with water. Why? So he'd be prepared for it if it happened during a race. Sure enough, that's exactly what happened at the 2008 Beijing Olympics. He overcame leaking goggles and took the gold medal.

When you embrace adversity and learn to adjust your frame of reference, you are able to build a life of resilience, adaptability, and appreciation. The great American writer and naturalist Henry David Thoreau spent two years living frugally in a small house in the woods so that he could "live deliberately, to front only the essential facts of life, and see if [he] could not learn what it had to teach."

Ask yourself: Could you live Spartan-like? Could you handle living a deliberate life? We're wired to do so. Our bodies are built for survival. Don't sit at home letting your life slip by and learning helplessness. Attack life. Test your limits. Search for a different frame of reference, and when you think you've gone far enough, go farther.

GET OFF THE COUCH!
How to Adjust Your Frame of Reference

Step 1. RECOGNIZE YOUR PESSIMISM. Your frame of reference is the context in which you view a situation. To change it, you first need to see it clearly for what it is. Identify your negativity. Explore your pessimism. Write down your negative thoughts and assumptions in a column on the left side of a sheet of lined paper. Review your list, and then add a column to the right where you write down the evidence to support that assumption. This should be easy to do; after all, you've already convinced yourself that you are right. Now, finally, to the right of your evidence, write down facts and comments that argue against your negative thought. This is going to be a lot harder, but it is where the growth comes in. You have to learn to convince yourself to change your mind using a compelling argument that changes your frame of reference. Once you can see how you have distorted reality with your negative thoughts, you change your frame of reference and are better able to see solutions to problems right before your eyes.

For example, let's say your boss reviews your report and sends a tersely worded note asking you to revise one section. You get defensive and tell a friend that the boss "hated" the report that you worked so hard on. "I suck at my job," you say. "I always screw up and the boss hates me."

Let's try to adjust your frame of reference by challenging those negative thoughts:

Column One (list the negatives)

1. Boss hates the report.

2. I suck, always screw up.

3. Boss hates me.

Column Two (list the support for your conclusions)

1. He wrote a terse note of criticism.

2. I've been asked to revise my work before.

3. Boss has criticized me before.

Column Three (argue against the negative)

1. Maybe I misinterpreted his tone of voice. After all, he asked for one small revision and actually thought the rest of the report was great.

2. Revising to make the work better is part of the learning process. Everyone needs an editor. If he didn't have confidence I could do the work, he would have revised it himself.

3. Criticizing part of my work doesn't mean he doesn't like me as an employee or a person. In fact, last month, he gave me a great quarterly review.

Challenging negative thoughts is one way to recognize when you are distorting the truth. By changing your frame of reference to a more realistic perspective, you can approach the challenge, in this case, revising the report, with a positive attitude that will lead to a better outcome.

You can use this kind of reframing exercise for any situation where your pessimistic instincts tell you things look bleak. Changing your frame of reference clears the fog of negativity between you and your True North.

Step 2. PRACTICE OPTIMISM by attacking the problem. Nothing good comes from negativity and self-doubt, so don't allow those thoughts to waste your time. Replace problem-focused thinking with solution-focused thinking. When faced with a roadblock, ask yourself: What's one thing I can do to make this situation better? Where's my work-around? By trying to solve the problem like a NASA engineer, you immediately sense yourself moving forward toward possibility and hope—the foundations of optimistic thinking.

Step 3. BUILD OBSTACLE IMMUNITY by deliberately creating adversity. Don't wait for adversity to test you. Make it happen. Remember how Michael Phelps's coach would deliberately break his swim goggles? Tiger Woods's dad would do something similar during practice sessions with his son. Instead of allowing Tiger to hit balls from a perfect lie, he would toss a bunch of balls on the grass and then step on them to press them into the turf to make them harder to hit. You can do the same by creating adverse situations in your life to force yourself out of your comfort zone. Here's some deliberate adversity to try:

Delayed Gratification Challenge:
- Skip dinner one day.
- Avoid alcohol for two weeks.
- Only buy food from farm stands this week.

- Eat meatless meals for one week.
- Fast for sixteen hours.

Technology Challenge:
o Turn off your cell phone for one week.
o Do not use any form of social media for a week.
o Unplug the television.
o Mow the lawn with a push mower.
o Build a fire without matches (using a flint and steel).
o Ride your bicycle to work or to the grocery store.

Exercise Challenge:
o Wake up at 5 a.m. to exercise.
o Do thirty burpees every day.
o Go for a hike wearing a backpack loaded with forty pounds of gear or several sandbags.
o Work out once in the morning and once in the evening daily for one week.
o Train for a classic one hundred-mile "century" bike ride.
o If you can't do a single pull-up, start by practicing a dead hang. Just grab a pull-up bar and hang as long as you can to build grip and arm strength. Then work up to doing one pull-up and then ten. Next build up to fifteen and so on.

Relationships Challenge:
o Take a day off in the middle of the week and do not check in with work.
o Never miss dinner with the family because of work.
o Take your wife on a date once a week.
o Call or hand-write a note to a different friend each week.
o Apologize to someone you have hurt or wronged.

○ Join an enthusiast club or service organization.
○ Volunteer at a soup kitchen or an assisted living facility.

Discomfort Challenge:
○ Take only cold showers.
○ Avoid sitting at work.
○ Sleep under the stars without a tent or sleeping bag.
○ Tread water, deadman float, or swim in a pool for an hour without touching bottom or holding on to the sides.
○ Hold your breath as long as you can.
○ Hold a plank for sixty seconds and then add ten seconds to the hold every day.
○ Sign up for a Spartan Race, a half marathon.

   Keep a journal of your adversity challenges, taking detailed notes about your experience and how changing your frame of reference has helped you to learn optimism.

PRINCIPLE #9

BE HONORABLE

The ultimate measure of a man is not where he stands in moments of comfort and convenience, but where he stands at times of challenge and controversy.
—MARTIN LUTHER KING, JR.

Ability without honor is useless.
—MARCUS TULLIUS CICERO

Integrity" stems from the Latin word *integer,* which means "soundness, wholeness, and completeness." It means to fully be who you are, authentic, consistent in your character, and visible in how you live your values. You don't wear masks. You don't behave like a friend one minute and an asshole the next. You don't talk about people behind their backs and you don't lie. I like this definition of integrity: doing the right thing all the time, even when no one is looking.

History is filled with stories of people with great integrity. I find them inspiring. Sometimes I wonder what I would do if I wore their shoes. Here are three favorite stories of integrity. I think they'll inspire you to be a better person, too.

The first goes back to World War II. In 1942, Irena Sendler, a Polish Catholic living in Warsaw, began smuggling children out of a sixteen-block area known as the Warsaw Ghetto. The ghetto was sealed. The Jewish families that had been forced to live behind its walls were dying from starvation and disease.

Sendler was a senior administrator in the Warsaw Social Welfare Department, and she managed to secure a pass into the ghetto, bringing food, medicines, and clothing to the desperate people living there. As the weekly death toll climbed, she decided she had to try to get the Jewish children out of the ghetto and on to safety.

In the twelve months between 1942 and 1943, Sendler helped 2,500 people escape. Some children were smuggled out in potato sacks. Some were carried out in body bags. Some were carried out in coffins. A mechanic took a baby out in his toolbox. Sendler and her brave recruits found non-Jewish families to adopt them using false identifications.

She kept the only record of their true identities in jars buried beneath an apple tree in a neighbor's backyard. She promised herself that one day when it was safe she would dig up the jars, locate the children, and inform them of their past.

In 1943, the Nazis became aware of her underground work and arrested her. Sendler was imprisoned and brutally tortured by the Gestapo. She was thrown into prison and left to die. But she never revealed the identity of the children and the families that took them in. Somehow, she survived. When the war ended, she tracked down as many of the children as she could and kept her promise to tell them what had happened and who they were.

The second comes more than thirty years later. In the mid-1970s, Apple and Microsoft were born, and they would change the world forever.

Their founders, Steve Jobs and Bill Gates, competed against one another for decades. Jobs disliked Gates. He accused him of ripping off other people's ideas, calling Gates unimaginative and Gates's products "third-rate."

"The only problem with Microsoft is they just have no taste," Jobs said in the 1996 public television documentary *Triumph of the Nerds.*

Gates mostly kept his opinions to himself. On occasion, he would respond with mild criticisms of his own. But he also praised Jobs for his immense contributions to the industry. In a 2012 interview, Gates talked about their so-called feud: "There was no peace to make. We were not at war. We made great products, and competition was always a positive thing. There was no [cause for] forgiveness."

The third story is more recent. In March 2011, a 9.9 magnitude earthquake off the eastern coast of Japan triggered a tsunami that crashed down on the Daiichi nuclear plant in Fukushima. You may recall that several of the reactors were severely damaged, causing the world's worst nuclear crisis since Chernobyl. Close to 20,000 people were killed, while 150,000 more were forced to evacuate, losing their homes.

A seventy-two-year-old man named Yasuteru Yamada decided he had to do something to help. He was a retired engineer who had spent his career building power plants. As he watched young workers dressed in HAZMAT suits report for nuclear cleanup duty, he felt compelled to take their place so they wouldn't be exposed to the radiation. He began calling up old colleagues and friends over the age of sixty who had relevant expertise. Within a couple of weeks close to five hundred retired men and women had volunteered to manage the cleanup in place of the younger generation.

Speaking to the press, Yamada explained that volunteering to take the place of younger workers was not altruistic or courageous but logical. The cells of an older person's body divide more slowly than a younger person's. He figured that by the time cancer from radiation set in most of the volunteers would have died of old age anyway. Volunteering to put themselves in the place of younger men was their duty.

Irena Sendler. Bill Gates. Yasuteru Yamada. What do these three different people whose life played out on three different continents have in common? What traits do they share that sets them apart from others? For me, one stands out over others: Honor.

Honor is about knowing what's right and following through. It is sticking with your values, regardless of the situation. The basis of honor is integrity, one of the most important of the Spartan virtues.

Threatened with death, Irena Sandler could not sacrifice the identity of those Jewish children she saved in order to save herself. Bill Gates could have met Jobs's taunts with his own, but instead chose to take the high road of integrity. Yasuteru Yamada placed duty to country and concern for younger men before his own safety. He was driven to volunteer by a burning sense of honor and responsibility, and he stoked those values in other men like him.

Integrity is a difficult principle to master. It's easy to compartmentalize integrity and be honorable part-time when it's convenient. Hell, often, we don't even recognize when we are being dishonorable. This usually happens when we unconsciously rationalize that our dishonesty isn't hurting anyone.

Check out this research that proves how easy it is to lie. A University of Massachusetts psychologist recruited 121 pairs of undergrads and asked them to have a conversation with another person. Some participants were asked to try to make themselves appear likable. Others were told to seem competent. The control group was not prompted at all. None of the groups were informed that the conversations would be monitored, but later they were told that they had been videotaped and were asked to watch the tapes and point out the false statements they made. It turned out that 60 percent of the college students lied. They told an average of two to three lies in just ten minutes.

Some lies were minor. For instance, agreeing with the other person when they really did not. Some were crazy, like falsely claiming to be a singer in a rock band. What's interesting is that men and women lied differently. Women tended to lie to make the person they were talking to feel good, while men lied to impress. "We didn't expect lying to be such a common part of daily life," said Robert S. Feldman, the author of the study and of the book *The Liar in Your Life.*

This study is fascinating to me because it demonstrates just how easy lying can be. We do it almost without thinking. Often, it's not malicious but simply the path of least resistance and pain. Or it's the easiest way to achieve what we want. That's why honor is so difficult and so worthwhile. Everyone wants to be known as having integrity. But it's elusive to most people because they neglect a fundamental principle here—consistency.

Being honorable isn't something you can switch on and off. Integrity isn't something you show on a case-by-case basis. Every day, you are presented with the choice to use it or not. Honor requires intentional thought and action. You have to make a choice. It's easy to forget that decision-making part when you're angry, stressed, or feeling afraid. So you mess up. You lash out. You act without thinking and, in doing so, you act without honor. You default to taking the path of least resistance.

Think about the last time you felt embarrassed for something you said or did in the heat of emotion. Maybe you flipped the middle finger to a driver who cut you off only to realize a split-second later that the driver was your daughter's second-grade teacher. *Shit!* Maybe you told your wife you had to work late when you really went to happy hour with the gang at the office and when she found out you got defensive and screamed at her that she's "too controlling." Have you ever taken credit for someone else's efforts or let someone at work take the blame for your screwup?

MASTER CLASS

Lewis Howes, author of THE SCHOOL OF GREAT-
NESS: A REAL-WORLD GUIDE TO LIVING BIGGER, LOVING
DEEPER, AND LEAVING A LEGACY

BEING HONORABLE

Create a Personal Principles Declaration, a statement of who you will be and what you will stand for in your life, even in the toughest moments. You will never achieve what you really want if you let your ego stand in the way of your principles. This is my Personal Principles Declaration:

Love myself, everyone, and everything.

Be in service to support others and the world.

Always give my best and strive for greatness in everything I do.

Live in abundance.

Create a win/win with everything.

Here's where mindfulness can save your reputation and, most important, your self-respect. Take a step back. Hit the pause button. Create a space of time between the stimulation and immediate action. Reflect on the choice at hand in the context of your core values. It's all about being more aware.

If you find it easy to regularly lie, your lack of integrity can chip away at other parts of your life and other behaviors. It's much harder to compromise your integrity if you are following your True North. When you commit to being authentic and to fulfilling your purpose, you learn to trust your conviction. And you'll start to feel uncomfortable whenever you begin to do something that may weaken others' trust in you. Integrity is a driver of trust.

Nothing compromises integrity like greed. History is littered with stories of people and organizations that acted without integrity. Bernie Madoff's enormous Ponzi scheme and the Lehman Brothers bankruptcy are two that come immediately to mind. CEOs overstate earnings to tell boards of directors and shareholders what they want to hear. Auto manufacturers cover up mistakes to avoid expensive recalls.

It's nice to share one story of greed that has a feel-good ending. Courtney and I were on our honeymoon with another couple who had also just married. I got called back to Wall Street because a company was interested in buying my firm. I felt terrible when I had to leave early—especially considering my friend was picking up the tab! But it was an offer I couldn't refuse, so I left my honeymoon about halfway through.

I met with these buyers. They had done their research. They determined that there were five or six guys at my firm who were responsible for 80 percent of our revenue. Instead of buying me out, they poached my staff. They offered these guys each $1 million a year. I didn't have a contract with these employees because they were *my guys*, friends from the old neighborhood who came to work for me.

There's an old saying that goes something like, "You don't truly know a person until you eat a barrel of salt with him." Well, I thought I knew these guys, and I just assumed they were loyal, but I guess I needed to eat more salt.

Then about two weeks after my guys left, one of them came to visit me. His nickname is "Socks" because when he first started working for me he didn't have good shoes. Socks handed me a check for $300,000. He said he couldn't pass up the opportunity to take that new job, but he felt an obligation to me. He wanted to repay me for the opportunity I gave him and the spot he put me in by leaving. That's integrity!

Socks had no legal obligation to me. He just wanted to do the right thing. And I'm sure that $300K turned into $3 million in reputation because word got around about what he did. We remain friends to this day.

While there are examples of lack of integrity everywhere from Capitol Hill to your workplace, from professional sports to your kids' Little League, there are also many, many examples of integrity all around you. You will find people like Socks who live the Spartan Core Virtues. People you can learn from. I interview people of extreme accomplishment for my Spartan Up! podcasts because they are also people of great integrity. Success and integrity are intertwined. I want to learn from these people. And you can, too.

If you want to practice being honorable and building the skills to live a life of integrity, try this exercise:

1. Think about the people you most admire. Make a list of these people. They may be people you know personally, family, friends, people at work, or in your community. Also, consider people you don't personally know: Sports heroes, politicians, entertainers, business people, authors, educators, spiritual leaders, and historical figures. Your list can be as long or as short as you'd like.

2. Now next to each name, write down the traits and qualities that you admire in that person. Some might include courage, reliability, compassion, conscience, fearlessness, conviction, responsibility, frugality, fairness, respect, commitment, loyalty, tolerance—the list goes on and on.

3. Finally, identify the three to five people whose character traits you would like to have. Write those character traits on an index card and refer to it whenever you have to make a choice that impacts your integrity.

Memorize your words of honor so they roll off your tongue. Turn them into a mantra. There's power in reciting mantras, codes of conduct, and mottos. One of the most famous codes of ethics is the Ten Commandments. Whether you're religious or not, you can appreciate the ethical reasoning for at least some of the laws on that list. Think about the Marine Corps motto *semper fidelis,* a Latin phrase meaning "always faithful" or "always loyal," which declares that Marines always do their duty to their Corps, their country, and their fellow Marines.

There's a reason the Boy Scouts of America requires Scouts to recite the twelve points of the Boy Scout Law at every meeting. *"A Scout is trustworthy, loyal, helpful, friendly, courteous, kind, obedient, cheerful, thrifty, brave, clean, and reverent."* The organization believes that rote recitation will ultimately lead to ingrained values that will turn boys into productive citizens.

There's a reason we welcome you into the Spartan community of millions who share common values, interests, and ideas by inviting you to adopt the Spartan Honor Pledge:

With a determined sense of responsibility, I pledge these
statements as my new normal.
I will follow my True North.
I will commit to what is important.
I will be ambitious and motivated in all that I do.
I will value my time.
I will make all my decisions by examining the upside and downside.

> *I will delay gratification.*
> *I will Grit it out.*
> *I will shift my frame of reference.*
> *I will live each day honoring my Spartan journey.*

My personal mantra is "nothing is ever going to be easy and failure is not an option." Whenever I face a decision about time, money, commitment, I rattle off my True North priorities and they guide me, too:

- Health first.

- Family second.

- Business third.

- Fun fourth.

Honor means not compromising your values, especially when no one is looking. The benefit of living honorably is enormous. When you act with integrity, you're also showing incredible respect for yourself, something on which you can't put a price tag. Author Steven Pressfield believes that self-respect and honor are inextricably linked, but they've become the exception rather than the norm. "We're starved of honor today in our culture," he says. "We prize the easy way to do anything, but what's missing is personal self-respect, where someone can say, 'Well, I'm actually engaged in an honorable pursuit.'"

My values are strongly tied up with the values of Spartan Race. I believe you have to try even if that sometimes means failing. You have to be accountable even when things go wrong. You have to challenge, push, to press on when things get hard, and even more when they get harder. You have to be brave enough to break and then stand back up again. Even

HONESTLY, GIVE A FUCK

It's hard to imagine honest Abe Lincoln flipping anyone the bird, but a new study analyzing profanity and honesty found a link between frequent swearing and trustworthiness. Researchers in the Netherlands conducted several studies that identified how frequently 276 individuals reported cursing and then gave those people a standard personality questionnaire that measured integrity. While cursing like a sailor is typically associated with moral turpitude, the study found that blurting out curse words is associated with forthrightness and authenticity, two characteristics of honesty and integrity.

though I have these values, they're only valuable if I can understand that others struggle with them. When I see participants without a limb or who are very overweight running one of our races, I need to be able to understand the difficulties they have in their lives and the race without believing I should compromise my values to "make it easier."

I spoke with Pressfield when I was writing my last book, "*Spartan Fit!*" He believes this lack of an honorable pursuit has left people distracted and disengaged with life, and I agree. The "cult of the individual," he says, has become more important than standing by a common code of ethics. But it's in this common code that honor lives. While putting yourself and your needs first can create a healthy form of individualism, idolizing the self can prompt a sense of self-interest, privilege, and victimhood. "The greatest thing in the world is to know how to belong to oneself," said French Renaissance writer Michel de Montaigne. I agree, but you also need to know how to share yourself. And sharing yourself, as Irena Sendler did, as Yasuteru Yamada did, and accepting that others' contributions can complement your own, as Bill Gates did, is a big part of being honorable. You do it, even when it's the difficult thing to do because you know it's right. And, in many ways, it makes things easier, because your choices come down to doing the thing that's right.

GET OFF THE COUCH!
How to Be Honorable

Step 1. BE CONFIDENT IN YOUR AUTHENTICITY. Build courage. Fear often keeps us from acting with honor and integrity. Fear and avoidance of the unpleasant creates ambiguity and indecision. Stand up for yourself and become comfortable saying "no." Be realistic: You can't say yes to everything and still honor your commitments. Be straightforward: People like to know where you stand.

Step 2. KEEP YOUR WORD. Fulfill your promises. Keep appointments. If you promise something, follow through. If you think you may not be able to commit, then don't. Integrity goes hand in hand with reliability.

Step 3. DO AN INTEGRITY CHECK. Honor is the quality of being fair, truthful, and sincere. When you are faced with a decision and you're unsure if your choice is honorable, ask yourself these questions to guide you:

1. Would I be willing to do this in front of my son, daughter, or someone else whose respect and opinion are important to me? (Often, we are dishonorable when no one is watching.)
2. Am I willing to speak my mind even though some may disagree or even ridicule me?
3. Am I passing the buck or am I taking responsibility?
4. Am I being unconditionally empathetic or is there something in it for me that is motivating me?

Step 4. ASSOCIATE WITH THE HONORABLE. Join communities that value integrity. Surround yourself with people you respect, read about and follow people who will influence your drive toward trustworthiness. Avoid people who lack integrity. Don't do business with them. Remember that people will inevitably judge your character by the character of your friends.

Step 5. RECRUIT AN HONESTY ACCOMPLICE. Be willing to have people police you. Ask a trusted friend, a co-worker or your spouse to give you honest feedback. Give that person a free pass to call you out when you are not living up to your expectations for yourself.

PRINCIPLE #10

BE SPARTAN

(SPARTAN VIRTUE: WHOLENESS)

If one advances confidently in the direction of his dreams, and endeavors to live the life, which he

has imagined, he will meet with a success unexpected in common hours.

—HENRY DAVID THOREAU

If we are facing in the right direction, all we have to do is keep on walking.

—ANCIENT BUDDHIST PROVERB

It's up to each one of us to summon what is within.

—DIANA NYAD

When you put the nine principles I've just laid out together, you'll find the tenth: Wholeness. You truly become Spartan.

One of the best examples of this is Diana Nyad. Over a period of almost thirty years, she attempted to swim between Cuba and Florida without a shark cage. Four times she failed.

On the fourth, at the age of sixty-three, she was attacked by a swarm of box jellyfish. I don't know if you know anything about box jellyfish. But if you do, you know why a swimmer might prefer to battle a shark.

Scientists named box jellyfish Cubozoa for their cube-shaped bell. But *sea wasp* is a much more appropriate name for these invertebrate bastards. Get this: They have fifteen tentacles up to ten-feet long, each containing five thousand stinging cells. Box jellyfish are considered the most toxic animal on the planet. Their venom is so painful a swimmer who is stung can go into shock and drown or die of a heart attack. Not only that, box jellyfish don't just float like most jellyfish do. They can swim after you.

Killer box jellies stung Diana Nyad during her fourth attempt and nearly killed her. She had to stop. She couldn't possibly continue. She later said that the stings made her feel as if her body had been "dipped in burning hot wax oil."

At that point, at age sixty-three, she might have given up on her dream, simply satisfied to have survived the last attempt. Not Nyad. Her unstoppable will drove her to learn what she could from the fourth failure and try a fifth time the following year.

On September 2, 2013, at the age of sixty-four, almost thirty years after her first attempt, she walked into the surf off Havana for a fifth time, repeating her mantra, *Find a way.* And she did. Fifty-three hours and 111 miles later, she became the first person to complete the open ocean swim from Havana to Key West without a shark cage.

Go on YouTube and watch her take the final steps to shore. You will see what is possible when you are Spartan.

How did Nyad weather four crushing failures and find the will to keep coming back? How did she endure storms, fatigue, hypothermia, vomiting, strong currents, sharks, and those killer sea wasps to reach her life's goal? When she struggled out of the water at Key West, she gave the crowd three answers:

1. Never, ever give up.

2. You're never too old to chase your dreams.

3. It looks like a solitary sport, but it's a team.

Nyad's record-setting swim was a triumph of the human spirit, one of the most remarkable feats of passion and endurance the world has ever witnessed. Her grit in the face of unbearable adversity blows me away, and at the same time I recognize the simplicity in her path to success. How did she do it? She identified her True North decades earlier and let nothing stop her from reaching it. In an interview a few years after her epic swim, she described herself as "just a person who cherishes a bold journey—who refuses to let this one wild and precious life slip quietly by."

"YOU'LL KNOW AT THE FINISH LINE."

What will you learn when you reach your Key West?

When people ask me, "Why do a Spartan Race?" my answer is, *"You'll know at the finish line."* It's our Spartan tagline. I'm deliberately vague because there's no single definitive answer to why anyone puts himself or herself through a course of manufactured hell or 10X hell, for that matter.

What you'll know at the finish line will be different from what your buddy or wife, or the stranger next to you will know. It's different for everyone who crosses the line. But that's what makes Spartan worthwhile. And cool. No matter how many races you enter, every step of the course is an opportunity to learn something new about *yourself.* I've heard it from thousands of people all over the world. One thing is certain though, and universal: You are a different person at the finish line. You have been transformed in some way that's unique to you. Do a race. You'll see.

You'll realize almost immediately that the transformation process begins long before you reach the start. When you sign up, you're a little bit different from the moment before you hit that send button. Every day you train, you change. You are different at the starting line than you were when you woke up that morning and drove to the course. Completing the Atlas Carry rewards you with something different than the Bucket Brigade and the Hercules Hoist challenges, and only you'll know what that is after you complete them. Sucking wind with cotton mouth and scraped knees at the finish line, you are different than you were hours earlier at the gun when you were fresh, your Camelbak was full of ice-cold water, and adrenaline was coursing through your veins in anticipation. At the finish line, you might be too freakin' exhausted to comprehend how you've changed or what you've learned. But the answer will come in time. And it will bring you back, looking for more answers.

BECOMING SPARTAN

Now, you've come to the finish line of this book. Have you changed? Have you seen how the path to your True North can deliver a fuller, richer, more satisfying life based on self-reliance and grit?

Like the pattern of obstacles in a Spartan Race, this book has guided you through the nine key principles of living the Spartan Life. Principle #10 is becoming Spartan, complete and whole, by pulling it all together, learning from your mistakes as Nyad did from hers, and engaging all the previous principles collectively into one unbeatable package.

The Spartan Way is your blueprint for living a successful life. If you mastered each of the ten Spartan principles by doing the exercises, soul searching, asking the hard questions, and practicing the strategies, then you will nail it. That doesn't mean you won't fail, hit snags, or face your own sea wasps. You will, but you'll have the tools to ride out the tough stuff and overcome. You won't become a prisoner to them.

I love what Dr. Maria Nemeth has to say about success. Maria Nemeth is a PhD, with about thirty years of experience as a clinical psychologist, and she wrote a fascinating book called *The Energy of Money: A Spiritual Guide to Financial and Personal Fulfillment.*

Nemeth defines success as "doing what you said you would do consistently with clarity, focus, ease, and grace." That's spot on. So good, let's look at those words again. *Doing what you said you would do consistently with clarity, focus, ease, and grace.* When you live the principles of *The Spartan Way,* that's exactly how you perform, with ease and grace, every day. When you possess clarity, you've discerned what's meaningful to you. It's your True North. Focus means you've turned your attention to what's important and committed to follow through, no matter what. Nemeth believes there's a great character distinction between people who are successful and those who are not. "It's being willing to do something even though you don't want to do it," she writes. "A pregnant woman does not want to go through the discomfort of childbirth, but she is *willing.*"

She is willing. That's what makes the difference. She's on that "desperate ground" that Sun Tzu wrote of in *The Art of War*—or a shark-infested ocean—that place where there are no options for retreating, where "officers and men alike will put forth their utmost strength."

"Being willing will change the course of your life," says Maria Nemeth.

I believe that. Unfortunately, I also believe we are becoming *the land of the unwilling.* Most people are unwilling to do, to try, to extend beyond the comfort of their couches and heated car seats. They are unwilling to do the hard stuff, even when they know the hard stuff is what's required for success. Look around you. We spend our lives avoiding discomfort, sweat, and struggle. We look for the shortcut, the easy route. How many times have you been taught to avoid the obstacles and seek the easier way?

It's been ingrained in us by our American culture. That's not the Spartan Way.

When my kids were very young, I signed them up for a race. They were in great shape and they could run fast. They sprinted off the starting line like Olympic champions but when they got to a mud puddle, they stopped dead in their tracks. They didn't know what to do. Why? Because, as we were all taught *you don't get your clothes dirty!*

Look, if we spend our lives in the gated community of our comfort zones, avoiding difficulty and obstacles, and mud puddles, what the hell will we do when we get some real shit thrown at us? How will we respond when we lose our job, our house, or our marriage? How will we react when a member of our family is diagnosed with cancer? We need to develop resilience and grit.

"An easy life is no life at all," declares Johnny Waite, our own master of human psychology, resident guru of obstacle immunity, and the Quality Manager for all Spartan Races. What's worse, he says, "by trying to avoid difficulty and failure we end up patterning failure, which is a dangerous trap. Instead, wish for a challenging life and the strength to do it."

Amen, brother.

When you embrace challenge and welcome adversity—even if it's manufactured adversity—you test the waters of resilience. You begin to develop discipline and grit and start to prepare yourself for the inevitable hardships down the road that have your name scrawled on them. And those hardships are there. They are coming your way. They are coming stealthily with ten-foot-long tentacles. But when you've faced true adversity before, the new problems will never seem as overwhelming. You won't freak, throw up your hands, and get emotional. You'll assess the problem, make some informed decisions, and get busy. There is another example I can come up with for this mindset.

Sir Ernest Henry Shackleton.

If you are new to Spartan Race, you may not be aware of him. But anyone who has come to compete knows why Shackleton is our hero. Shackleton was a fearless British polar explorer, whose grit and fortitude inspires all of us. He made two failed attempts to become the first man to reach the South Pole. A Norwegian explorer beat him to the goal in 1911. But disappointment didn't deter Shackleton. In 1914, he devised another challenge, to become the first man to cross Antarctica, from end to end, through the South Pole.

He would take two ships. Shackleton's would cross the treacherous Weddell Sea and land at Vahsel Bay. A supply ship would sail the Ross Sea and deliver food for the overland leg of the trip. The journey was daunting and success was unlikely. The Weddell Sea was notorious for crushing ice floes and the route was uncharted. Shackleton didn't downplay the dangers in his recruitment advertisement, which read:

MEN WANTED

FOR HAZARDOUS JOURNEY. SMALL WAGES, BITTER COLD.

LONG MONTHS OF COMPLETE DARKNESS, CONSTANT DANGER, SAFE RETURN

DOUBTFUL. HONOR AND RECOGNITION

IN CASE OF SUCCESS.

ERNEST SHACKLETON

Five thousand men answered the advertisement. Fifty-six were chosen as Shackleton's crew, and they set sail. Shackleton skippered a three-hundred-ton schooner aptly named *Endurance* in honor of his family motto *fortitudine vincimus* ("By endurance we conquer.")

For six weeks, *Endurance* had sailed more than twelve thousand miles through frozen seas. The next one thousand miles, the ship pushed through giant slabs of pack ice, some thrusting twenty feet in the air. Then, one hundred miles from its destination, *Endurance* became trapped, stuck motionless in the ice. Eventually, the ice began to press on the ship and crush it. The men abandoned *Endurance* on Shackleton's orders and set up "Ocean Camp" using the ship's broken timbers for shelter. *Endurance* eventually sank in October 1915.

Six months later, the sea ice melted enough for the men to pile into the three surviving lifeboats and take to the sea for Elephant Island, about a hundred miles away. They had little food left. After seven days of enduring storms and cold in the open boats, they arrived barely alive on the uninhabited island.

Shackleton knew rescue was impossible; they were marooned too far from the trade lanes at sea. So he and five volunteers set one of the lifeboats into the sea again, this time in hopes of reaching whaling camps off South Georgia Island over eight hundred miles away. The attempt became one of the most epic sea journeys of all time—seventeen days of tossing on the planet's stormiest oceans through hurricane-force winds and waves twenty-feet high. They made land but then had to traverse twenty-two miles over glacier-covered mountains to reach help. Three attempts to return to Elephant Island failed, but on the fourth, Shackleton rescued his men. All twenty-eight survived.

The Shackleton story resonates with Spartans for many reasons. For one, it was a feat of incredible endurance and survival under the most brutal weather conditions. It provides perspective when we face our own, much milder challenges. Second, the journey shows the depth of Shackleton's character and his integrity. He never lost his composure despite all these frustrating failures. He led the men through each setback with stoic resolve. He was committed to those men who devoted their lives to his quest. While hiking toward the whaling camps, he told his rescue crew, "If anything happens to me while those fellows are waiting for me, I shall feel like a murderer."

Shackleton embodies the principles of the Spartan Way. He was a common man, not an aristocrat, but a man who lived his life in an earthy, straightforward way. He knew what he wanted—his True North—and he strived to get it. He never gave up or put himself before his men, and as result he won the admiration of a country and the devotion of those who followed him. Shackleton was not perfect, he made many mistakes, but he was a whole man who loved life and inspired others to strive to achieve the impossible. Perhaps his greatest genius was his ability to be optimistic in dire situations, realistic about his options, and intuitive about what he needed to do to move forward.

THE BATTLE IN YOUR MIND

Like Shackleton and Nyad, elite warriors know that to win on the real battlefield, you must first win on the battlefield of your mind. This requires mastering your emotions, not getting caught up in fear, worry, and indecision. Those things destroy confidence. On the surface, a Spartan Race may seem to be about physical strength and endurance, but the ultimate goal, as you've learned through *The Spartan Way,* is to build mental strength. The value of an obstacle race is that it forces you to live in the moment, to focus completely on getting through the challenge without thinking about past or future—only the present, the barbed wire before you. You can't worry about making a mortgage payment when your legs are cramped with lactic acid and you can't suck enough oxygen into your lungs. Breathing trumps money worries in that instant. If for only an hour or two you are completely free of anything else you think may matter in your life, you've won the race. You are experiencing the life-altering power of *obstacle immunity.*

Something else beneficial happens as you build up your immunity to adversity: You realize that challenge and struggle produce offspring with names like confidence, adaptability, vitality, tenacity, exuberance, and joy.

Czikszentmihalyi, the psychologist I mentioned earlier who coined the concept of flow, wrote about struggle: "Contrary to what we usually believe, moments like these, the best moments in our lives, are not the passive, receptive, relaxing times—although such experiences can also be enjoyable if we have worked hard to attain them. The best moments usually occur when a person's body or mind is stretched to its limits in voluntary effort to accomplish something difficult and worthwhile. Optimal experience is thus something that we can make happen."

We *can* make it happen. You *are* making it happen in your life right now by living the principles of the Spartan Way every day.

TRUE HONOR

I want to leave you with another story of Shackleton-esque integrity and Nyad-like grit that still gives me chills when I think about it. It comes out of one of the Death Races a few years back. It's about a woman I hold in high regard. Her name is Amy Palmiero-Winters. I'll set it up for you:

A Death Race is a brutal sixty-plus-hour event that takes place in the unexpectedly challenging terrain of the Green Mountains in and around Pittsfield, Vermont. There's no support, but there are emergency medical personnel on hand in case you're woefully injured. We don't tell you when it starts or ends, but we try to make you fail and quit every step of the way. Some people think it's pure insanity.

One section of this challenge is a mile swim in a frigid reservoir. After you complete the swim, you climb onto a floating dock. Surprise! There's a spinning wheel set up like the ones you see down on the boardwalk for winning stuffed animals. Instead of plush toys, the prize here is being forced

WHAT I'VE LEARNED

Amy Palmiero-Winters, mother of two, welder, the first athlete with a prosthetic leg to complete the 100-mile Western States Endurance Run, and a member of Team Step Ahead, a group of elite disabled athletes

When the doctors told me they had to remove my leg (I was in a motorcycle accident), I had to take the only option I was given and make the best of it. I realized I had been given a second chance at life to get up, do, and be my absolute best.

The purpose of the Spartan Race is to pull out the best in people without having them go through something traumatic like losing a leg. The race will push you like you've never been pushed, but it'll make you stronger. It's life-changing. It's energizing.

I love obstacle racing because it gives me the opportunity to help others see what's possible in their lives. Scars don't dictate who we are, but they can build incredible strength within us.

to get back in the water for more swimming. Just one sliver of pie on that Wheel of Fortune says, "You're done swimming." If the ticker ends up on any other sliver, you're back in the water for another mile swim.

When you're exhausted, shivering, and half-drowned, your mind plays tricks on you. For some unknown reason, while swimming, you're convinced that the next wheel spin is going to stop on "you're done swimming." You can't fathom having to jump back in the water . . . again.

Amy and two six-foot-tall, rock-hard Marines climbed onto the dock and spun the wheel to learn their fate. Would they have to swim a third frigid mile? You know where this is going. The wheel read "back in the water!" But, hold on, it was worse than that. All three were officially disqualified from the race for not making the time cut-off for the mile-swim challenge. "You're out. Go home," I told them.

Amy was forty-two at the time and an amputee. She lost her left leg below the knee as a result of a motorcycle accident. While she was sitting there dumping the lake water out of her prosthetic lower leg, the two young Marines broke down on the dock. Physically and mentally spent, they started complaining, moaning, and even crying about being disqualified.

I used a few choice words to get those crybabies off the dock so the EMTs could tend to Amy who was hypothermic. But here's what really surprised me: A half hour later, with some of the color back in her face, Amy strapped her prosthesis back on and said, "Joe, I know I'm officially out, but I'm here and I want to finish the race. What do you say?"

What *do* I say to that? How do I respond to someone who is so fucking badass, she wants more torture even though she's already failed?

I was thinking of Shackleton on that ice. I told her, "If you can get to *this* point by *this* time, you can go on. Not official."

She made it to the place on time. But that's not the end of the story. The next leg was an eighteen-mile mountain hike. I put her with a group of guys and told everyone they had to stick together as a team and look out for one another. They were all exhausted, muddy, and bloody. Some looked like they were sleepwalking.

Three hours later, I drove ahead to the next checkpoint and, miraculously, saw these guys coming out of the woods. I thought, "Wow, they must have been hoofing it." Then, I noticed that Amy was missing along with one big military guy with red hair. I think his name was Ben. "Why did the group break up?" I wondered. "They should have stayed together." I waited there. A couple of hours later, I saw redheaded Ben hike in with

Amy. I asked him what happened. He wouldn't look at me but just kept moving. Badass Amy didn't say a thing, either. She just moved on to the next segment, determined to crush it, *unofficially*.

Later, I learned that those bums who came in early cheated. They hopped in a mini van and took a shortcut. But Ben did all eighteen miles helping Amy, and neither of them ratted out those other guys. Man, when I think of integrity, I see a big redheaded guy and a woman with a prosthetic leg who just hiked eighteen brutal miles and kept a secret. Like I said, the story still gives me chills.

At the finish line, seconds to go before cutoff, Amy came sprinting in on two legs, one high tech, one flesh-and-blood, both muddy. "Oh my God, you're my hero," I told her.

Much later, I asked her why she didn't mention those guys who cheated. "It would have been a waste of energy," she said, "and you need every ounce of energy in a Death Race. Besides, those guys have to live with themselves knowing they cut corners. I went the distance and won the real prize."

How do *you* go the distance? The same way—by not cutting corners but embracing adversity and powering through it. The "real prize" of living the Spartan Way is the confidence and the satisfaction you'll gain every day simply by practicing these ten principles and grabbing the little wins that are stepping-stones to your True North. That's your blueprint for success. And Diana Nyad summed it up perfectly with four simple words:

NEVER, EVER GIVE UP.

LIVE THE SPARTAN WAY

A Spartan pushes his or her mind and body to the limit.

I am Spartan.

A Spartan masters his or her emotions.

I am Spartan.

A Spartan gives generously.

I am Spartan.

A Spartan leads.

I am Spartan.

A Spartan stands up for his or her beliefs no matter the cost.

I am Spartan.

A Spartan knows his or her flaws and strengths.

I am Spartan.

A Spartan proves himself through actions, not words.

I am Spartan.

A Spartan lives every day as if it were his or her last.

I am Spartan.

APPENDIX

SPARTAN HONOR PLEDGE

With a determined sense of responsibility, I pledge these statements:

I will follow my True North,

I will commit to what is important,

I will be ambitious and motivated in all that I do,

I will value my time,

I will make all my decisions by examining the upside and downside,

I will delay gratification,

I will grit it out,

I will shift my frame of reference,

I will live each day honoring my journey to live the Spartan Way.

Signature: _____

Date:_____

STRONG HABITS

28 Practices for Living the Spartan Life

Habits are powerful things. Bad habits are like a riptide that pulls you out to sea. They make it so much harder to reach your goals. Good habits bring you closer and closer to your goal.

Below are twenty-eight good habits that support the Spartan lifestyle. Take some time to work them into your life. The more positive the reward, the more closely tied it is to an important goal or dream, the more you'll want to repeat this cycle.

1. Take a cue to stand. If you have a desk job, do your back a favor and get in the habit of standing as much as possible at work. Get yourself a stand-up desk or, at least, use cues to remind you to stand every half hour. Set a timer on your computer or stand up every time you receive a phone call.

2. Make push-ups harder with a sandbag. Place a sandbag on the ground to your right. Assume a push-up position next to it. Do a push-up, then grab the sandbag with your left hand and drag it underneath you forcefully until it's now on your left side. Do another push-up and drag it back with your right hand. Keep it up for twenty reps.

3. Drink water, not juice. You may have heard that most of us are walking around dehydrated. That's debatable. But the fact is drinking water is preferable to drinking anything else, especially soda, alcohol, and fruit juice. Drinking enough water daily can help with weight management, skin health, and keeping your body efficient. Make a habit of walking around with a water bottle full of ice water. It's a good way to ensure you drink between sixty-four and ninety ounces of water per day, which most experts say is a good goal. Remember that milk, decaf coffee, and teas count toward your quota, and you do get water from many of the foods you eat. Your pee is a good gauge of whether you are drinking enough water. It should be the color of pale lemonade.

4. Practice deep breathing. A lot of people, especially older folks and the out-of-shape crowd, "chest breathe." In other words, they don't fully fill their lungs. Short chest breaths elevate anxiety. To develop good relaxation skills learn to "belly breathe." Take a deep breath so that your belly rises before your chest does. That's belly breathing, also known as diaphragmatic breathing. Practice five deep breaths before you go to bed, when you wake up, and several times throughout the day at work. When you feel stress rising, you'll have a well-practiced technique for calming your anxiety and channeling your focus.

5. Outsmart a rival at work. Never whine. Ever. But do communicate with the boss, proactively. When your boss dreams up a new project or seems under the gun, volunteer. You're not kissing ass if you do the work. You're working. And whether or not it ices out your rival, the important thing is that it advances the company's goals. And you'll feel good about that. Not only that, but your boss will notice that you're proactive.

6. Take a cold shower. I love 'em. Okay, no I don't. But I take them. German researchers found that cold baths increased disease-fighting white blood cells, improved circulation, and boosted testosterone for those who took them regularly. Plus, cold showers and baths are a terrific way to develop grit.

7. Run barefoot on the beach. Running on soft sand strengthens your calves, arches, and Achilles tendons and restores proper mechanics to flat-footed runners. It toughens up the bottom of your feet so you can advance to barefoot running on turf and dirt.

8. Seek out silence. Our world is too noisy. We need to experience quiet as much as possible. Gordon Hempton, a sound-recording artist known as the Sound Tracker, has been pursuing rare nature sounds for thirty-five years—sounds that can only be appreciated in the absence of man-made noise. One of the best ways to reduce stress, he says, is listening to the hum of insects at dawn. "Our ears are essentially animal ears, hundreds of thousands of years old and naturally tuned to the sounds of a fertile, healthy environment. So going into nature and listening is much more than an activity. In a way, it's also a homecoming."

9. Work out the first thing in the morning. I've been doing this for years. I get my exercise done before most people wake up. That way I never miss a workout. Apparently, working out in the morning gives you a better workout. Get this: A British study found that people who exercised at 6:45 a.m. pushed themselves harder and longer than people who worked out at 6:45 p.m.

10. Bored of burpees? Do 20 kettlebell swings. You'll be happy to return to burpees. Place a kettlebell on the floor. Stand over it with your feet spread slightly wider than shoulder width. Bend at the waist, pushing your hips back and grab the handle with both hands. Hike the bell between your legs and then thrust your hips forward as you swing the bell to chest level. Swing it back between your legs with a controlled motion (that makes it harder). Do twenty reps without stopping. University of Wisconsin researchers found that kettlebell swings properly done burn about fourteen calories per minute, about the same amount as running six miles an hour.

11. Rearrange your fridge. Move all your produce to eye level. According to Cornell University researchers, you're 2.7 times more likely to eat healthy food if it's in your line of sight.

12. Team up. It's easier to stay committed to your promise when you share that commitment with a partner or team. Think about it: It's 5:30 a.m. on a cold, drizzly morning and you're contemplating either going for a three-mile run or staying under the covers for another hour. You are more likely to jump out of bed if a friend or friends are waiting for you at the park in the rain. Friends keep friends accountable.

13. Nourish your neurons. Just fifteen to twenty minutes of cardio a day can lower Alzheimer's risk, according to Gary Small, MD, coauthor of *The Alzheimer's Prevention Program.* Increased blood flow helps brain cells communicate better, he says.

14. Do this when you screw up. Look him or her in the eye and say, "I messed up. I'm sorry." Then shut up. Your brevity shows remorse, respect, and sincerity. And it keeps you from rambling into excuses. As your grandfather used to say, "Honesty is the best policy."

15. Check the label. The best foods for your body don't come in boxes or cans. For those foods you need to buy packaged, check the nutrition facts label first. If the ingredient list is long and full of words you can't pronounce, feed it to the squirrels.

16. Grab an apple, take a walk. Instead of having a big lunch, take a brisk thirty-minute walk. Reward yourself with a piece of fruit at the end. Even a moderately paced walk for only thirty minutes per day can lower your risk for heart disease, according to cardiologists at the American Heart Association.

17. Have a smoothie with pea protein. People who eat processed meats have a higher risk of death than those who get their protein from plant sources, according to Harvard researchers. An easy way to replace meat protein is by making a smoothie with plant-based protein powder, such as pea protein. A Harvard study found that for every 3 percent increase in protein from plant sources, there was a reduction in risk of death by 10 percent.

18. Pick up heavy objects. Every decade after age thirty, men and women lose 3 to 5 percent of their muscle mass, a natural process called sarcopenia, due to a reduction in testosterone. To counteract muscle shrinking, do strength-training exercise every week. Resistance exercises, like weight lifting and bodyweight calisthenics, build lean muscle mass, which increases resting metabolic rate, protects joints, improves balance, and even improves bone density.

19. Be mindful, remember more. In a study reported in *Psychological Science,* college students who practiced mindfulness—awareness of the moment—for two weeks showed memory improvements. Mindfulness is the practice of purposely paying attention to the present moment nonjudgmentally in a way that invites insight. Try it tonight while doing something as mundane as washing the dinner dishes. Focus on the warmth of the water, the scent of the soap, the feel of the fork tines that just bit into your fingers, all the sights, sounds, and feelings of the experience. One study found that people who washed dishes mindfully, reported 27 percent less anxiety and a 25 percent increase in mental inspiration.

20. Exercise in the morning in a fasted state. Studies have shown that exerting yourself when you haven't eaten anything for eight hours or more, forces your body to tap into your fat stores for energy.

21. Keep a food diary. Training yourself to be a mindful eater is one of the best ways to lose weight and adopt healthier eating habits. A University of Arkansas study found that people who keep a food log for at least three weeks lost three and a half pounds more than people who didn't track their food intake.

22. Do more things you suck at. You'll help grow new brain connections. Can't sing? Keep trying. A mess at chess? Challenge the kids. Doing things that you aren't very accomplished at is a way of stepping out of your confort zone and growing—in skills and brain cells.

23. Get to sleep faster. Drink six ounces of tart cherry juice before going to bed. Tart cherries contain natural melatonin, the hormone that regulates sleep. And the carbohydrates in the juice increase the production of serotonin, which is a calming brain chemical that can help you fall asleep. Also, do what I do: Sleep cold. Turn down the heat. Kick off the heavy blanket. Lowering core body temperature helps induce sleep. Keep your bedroom cool, about sixty-five degrees or cooler. Another trick that works well in wintertime, especially in Vermont: Wear socks to bed. Warming feet causes blood vessels in your body to enlarge, allowing more heat to escape your body, which lowers your body temperature.

24. Take a stretch break. Once an hour, take a stretch break from work. Stand facing a corner of the room with your feet together about two feet back from the corner. Place your forearms on each wall, with your elbows slightly below shoulder height. Keep your head neutral, tucking your chin back slightly. Inhale and pull your abdominal muscles into your spine. Exhale and lean into the wall. You'll feel your shoulder blades squeeze together. Hold the stretch for five to thirty seconds and then return to the starting position. Repeat five times.

25. Grow your gut biome. Instead of a 10 a.m. coffee break, drink a glass of kefir, a fermented drink made from cow, goat, or sheep milk. It contains enzymes, yeasts, and probiotics, plus high levels of vitamin B_{12}, calcium, and magnesium and has been shown to heal "leaky gut" syndrome, inflammatory bowel disease, and boost the immune system.

26. Sweat outside. If you have a choice of exercising indoors or outdoors, always choose to get outside. A recent study at University of California San Diego found that people who exercised outdoors were more active and completed about thirty minutes more exercise each week than people who exercised indoors.

27. Lower your blood pressure. Have it checked every year. If it's high, that is above 120/80 mmHg, work with your doctor to get it down. High systolic blood pressure limits the brain of blood and nutrients, making it more likely that you will lose gray matter in critical areas as you age.

28. Learn a handful of amazing recipes for cooking salmon. Salmon, tuna, and other oily fish are rich in omega-3 fatty acids, which are important for all-around brain and heart health. Omega-3 fatty acids contain

DHA and EPA, which are highly concentrated in the brain and are crucial for optimal brain function, according to the Academy of Nutrition and Dietetics. These fatty acids are so important to consume because our neurons use them to build brain cell walls and maintain good brain health. In fact, people with low blood levels of omega-3s had lower brain volumes than people with higher levels, suggesting their brains were aging more rapidly. One study at Tufts University found that people who ate oily fish three times a week reduced their risk of Alzheimer's disease by nearly 40 percent.

GET SHIT DONE! PLANNER TEMPLATES

HEY (YOUR NAME HERE) GET SHIT DONE!	
MY TRUE NORTH:	
For the week of:	
Big Idea Goal: (Ambition) Linked to your True North	
This week's goal: (Motivation)	
This week's Small Steps:	
Monday	
Tuesday	
Wednesday	
Thursday	
Friday	
Saturday	
Sunday	
This week's Little Wins:	
Monday	
Tuesday	
Wednesday	
Thursday	
Friday	
Saturday	
Sunday	
How do you feel?	

HEY (YOUR NAME HERE) GET SHIT DONE!

MY TRUE NORTH:	
For the week of:	
Big Idea Goal: (Ambition) Linked to your True North	
This week's goal: (Motivation)	
This week's Small Steps:	
Monday	
Tuesday	
Wednesday	
Thursday	
Friday	
Saturday	
Sunday	
This week's Little Wins:	
Monday	
Tuesday	
Wednesday	
Thursday	
Friday	
Saturday	
Sunday	
How do you feel?	

HEY (YOUR NAME HERE) GET SHIT DONE!

MY TRUE NORTH:	
For the week of:	
Big Idea Goal: (Ambition) Linked to your True North	
This week's goal: (Motivation)	
This week's Small Steps:	
Monday	
Tuesday	
Wednesday	
Thursday	
Friday	
Saturday	
Sunday	
This week's Little Wins:	
Monday	
Tuesday	
Wednesday	
Thursday	
Friday	
Saturday	
Sunday	
How do you feel?	

HEY (YOUR NAME HERE) GET SHIT DONE!

MY TRUE NORTH:	
For the week of:	
Big Idea Goal: (Ambition) Linked to your True North	
This week's goal: (Motivation)	
This week's Small Steps:	
Monday	
Tuesday	
Wednesday	
Thursday	
Friday	
Saturday	
Sunday	
This week's Little Wins:	
Monday	
Tuesday	
Wednesday	
Thursday	
Friday	
Saturday	
Sunday	
How do you feel?	

HEY (YOUR NAME HERE) GET SHIT DONE!

MY TRUE NORTH:	
For the week of:	
Big Idea Goal: (Ambition) Linked to your True North	
This week's goal: (Motivation)	
This week's Small Steps:	
Monday	
Tuesday	
Wednesday	
Thursday	
Friday	
Saturday	
Sunday	
This week's Little Wins:	
Monday	
Tuesday	
Wednesday	
Thursday	
Friday	
Saturday	
Sunday	
How do you feel?	

ACKNOWLEDGMENTS

I'd like to thank the following people, without whose support and inspiration this book could not have been written.

My awesome wife and family who have put up with my insanity for years . . . all in an effort to help change the world, and also Spartan staff, Jay Jackson, Joe Wein, Jeff Csatari, Siobhan Colgan, Richard Branson, Barry Sternlicht, Jorge Lemann, Vinny Viola, Alan Jope, Cal Fussman, Barry Hearns, Dan Pena, Tony Robbins, General Stanley A. McChrystal, Tim Ferriss, Simon Whitfeld, and Theo Epstein.

I'd also like to thank the Capuccis for keeping me on track and Marion Abrams for her support with the Spartan Up! podcast, which helped to inform the content of this book.

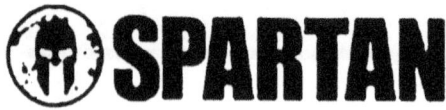

🛡️ SPARTAN

Joe De Sena
Founder and CEO, Spartan

Joe De Sena—founder and CEO of Spartan, the world's largest obstacle race and endurance brand—has demonstrated his entrepreneurial drive since his preteens. After building a multimillion-dollar pool and construction business in college, and creating a Wall Street trading firm, De Sena set his sights on ripping 100 million people off their couches by creating the Spartan lifestyle.

Following a successful career on Wall Street, De Sena moved his family to Pittsfield, Vermont, to operate an organic farm, a bed and breakfast, and a general store for hikers. It was here his passion grew for ultramarathons, adventure races, and endurance events, and thus the idea for Spartan was born.

With more than 1 million annual global participants at more than 200 events across more than 30 countries, Spartan offers heats for all fitness levels and ages, from beginner to elite and kids as young as four-year-olds. The brand has transformed more than 5 million lives since it was founded in 2010.

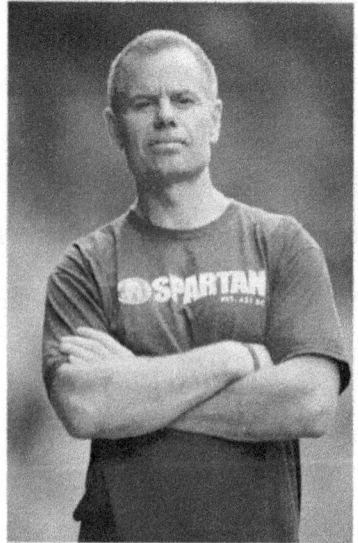

De Sena is also the *New York Times* bestselling author of *Spartan Up!* and *Spartan Fit!* As a popular keynote speaker, De Sena has parlayed the teachings of his Spartan principles into the SpartanX Leadership Forum, a series of events in which participants collaborate to solve challenges alongside business leaders while learning to overcome mental and physical obstacles.

In addition to race events, the Spartan lifestyle that De Sena built encompasses all the tools one needs to transform their lives, including partnerships with fitness brands such as Life Time, 24 Hour Fitness, and the Daily Burn; complementary training, nutrition plans, and content; television series on NBC and Facebook; forthcoming documentaries about the brand, sport, and health; and an extensive line of apparel and licensed fitness gear and equipment.

Throughout his lifetime, Joe has competed in any extreme sports adventure he could find, testing his mental and physical endurance against nature. Joe turned an interest in endurance racing into a passion. His racing resume is the stuff of legend—over 50 ultra-events overall and 14 Ironman events in one year alone.

Jeff Csatri is a *New York Times* bestselling author and former executive editor of *Men's Health* magazine.

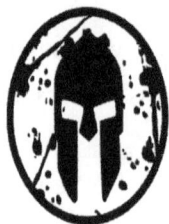

SPARTAN™

The Races

Spartan Sprint
Featuring 20 to 25 obstacles along 3 to 5 miles of terrain, the Spartan Sprint is the brand's shortest distance race and a favorite among new and returning racers. It's the perfect distance for thos looking to start their Spartan journey, allowing racers a manageable distance to test their limits.

Spartan Super
With 25 to 30 obstacles along 8 to 10 miles of terrain, the Spartar Super is the brand's middle-distance race. The event offers racers true athletic test that is an ideal blend of distance and speed.

Spartan Beast
With 30 to 35 obstacles along 12 to 14 miles of rugged terrain, th Spartan Beast tests everything competitors are made of: strength, endurance, and resolve. The event pushes competitors deep into their discomfort zones, and well past those self-imposed obstacle once considered limits.

More than just a race, Spartan also offers a wide range of training and educational programs for all levels.

To sign up for your first race, or to learn more, please visit www.spartan.com.

www.ingramcontent.com/pod-product-compliance
Lightning Source LLC
Chambersburg PA
CBHW021618270326
41931CB00008B/752